An Atlas of
OSTEOPOROSIS
Second Edition

THE ENCYCLOPEDIA OF VISUAL MEDICINE SERIES

An Atlas of
OSTEOPOROSIS
Second Edition

John C. Stevenson, FRCP, FESC

Rosen Laboratories of the Wynn Institute, Endocrinology and Metabolic Medicine,
Imperial College School of Medicine, London, UK

and

Michael S. Marsh, MD, MRCOG

Department of Obstetrics
King's College Hospital, London, UK

Foreword by
Robert Lindsay, MD

Helen Hayes Hospital
West Haverstraw, New York, USA

The Parthenon Publishing Group

International Publishers in Medicine, Science & Technology

NEW YORK   LONDON

Library of Congress Cataloging-in-Publication Data

Stevenson, John C. (John Curtis)
    An atlas of osteoporosis / John C. Stevenson and Michael S.
Marsh : foreword by Robert Lindsay. -- 2nd ed.
        p. cm. -- (The encyclopedia of visual medicine series)
    Includes bibliographical references and index.
    ISBN 1-85070-987-4
    1. Osteoporosis Atlases. I. Marsh, M. S. (Michael S.)
II. Title. III. Series.
    [DNLM: 1. Osteoporosis Atlases. WE 17 S847a 1999]
RC931.O73S78 1999
616.7'16--dc21
DNLM/DLC   99-35361
for Library of Congress   CIP

British Library Cataloguing in Publication Data

Stevenson, John C. (John Curtis)
    An atlas of osteoporosis. - 2nd ed. - (The encyclopedia of visual
medicine series)
    1. Osteoporosis
    I. Title II. Marsh, M.S. (Michael S.)
    616.7'16
    ISBN 1-85070-987-4

Published in the USA by
The Parthenon Publishing Group Inc.
One Blue Hill Plaza
PO Box 1564, Pearl River
New York 10965, USA

Published in the UK and Europe by
The Parthenon Publishing Group Limited
Casterton Hall, Carnforth
Lancs. LA6 2LA, UK

Copyright ©2000 Parthenon Publishing Group

Printed and bound in Spain by
T.G. Hostench, S.A.

Contents

Foreword

Over the last several years, many volumes have appeared on the subject of osteoporosis. Most of these are multi-authored books with a high degree of scientific accuracy, but the usual heterogeneity in writing style. In this, the second edition of *An Atlas of Osteoporosis*, Drs Stevenson and Marsh have produced an exciting volume that provides cogent evaluation of the pathophysiology, prevention and treatment of osteoporosis, together with a large number of figures and diagrams. This unique approach to osteoporosis provides a valuable resource for physicians who practice in the field and for those who see patients with osteoporosis only occasionally, but particularly for young physicians as they enter their career. Written in a readable style throughout, the many illustrations enhance the text, fulfiling the old adage, 'a picture is worth a thousand words'. Of particular importance are the images surrounding the techniques of bone densitometry, which demonstrate not only the techniques, but the output from the techniques. This provides an introduction for the practicing physician to the technology which is gradually becoming of increasing clinical importance. Osteoporosis is now defined as a disease of low bone density. Thus, in order to make the diagnosis, the clinician has to make use of the investigative procedure of bone densitometry. However, many physicians are still wary of a test that they did not learn about in medical school or during their early training. This volume places that test in its clinical context, provides a review of a majority of the tests that are currently available and should enhance the comfort level of any practicing physician with this investigation. In situations in which the original print-outs are not provided to the practicing doctor from the densitometry unit, the illustrations here allow the clinician to provide simple explanation to the patient about the test, its meaning, its interpretation and its clinical utility.

The senior author, Dr John Stevenson, is a Reader in Medicine at Imperial College and is an international expert in the field of osteoporosis and metabolic medicine. In this volume, Dr Stevenson brings his outstanding gifts as a teacher and scientist and provides the high-quality, factual information required to make a success of this volume. He is ably supported by Dr Michael Marsh who is an obstetrician/gynecologist with a thorough understanding of this disease and its importance for the Ob/Gyn community. In this second edition, they have enhanced figures, updated and revised text, and provide a detailed account of the advances that have occurred in osteoporosis in a format of particular use to clinicians. I can thoroughly recommend this book to those with both a passing and a detailed interest in this disease.

Dr Robert Lindsay
Helen Hayes Hospital
West Haverstraw
New York, USA

Acknowledgements

The authors are grateful to the following colleagues who so kindly provided some of the illustrations included in this atlas:

Mr Paul R. Allen, Consultant Orthopaedic Surgeon, Bromley Hospital, London;

Ms Linda Banks, Superintendent Radiographer, Royal Postgraduate Medical School, London;

Professors Alan Boyde and *Sheila Jones*, and *Mr J.A.P. Jayasinghe*, Hard Tissue Research Unit, Department of Anatomy and Developmental Biology, University College, London;

Dr David Dempster and *Professor Robert Lindsay*, Regional Bone Center, Helen Hayes Hospital, West Haverstraw, New York;

Dr Belinda Lees, Clinical Trials and Evaluation Unit, Royal Brompton Hospital, London;

Dr Flemming Melsen, University Department of Pathology, Aarhus County Hospital, Aarhus, Denmark

Dr Leif Mosekilde, University Department of Endocrinology and Metabolism, Aarhus County Hospital, Aarhus, Denmark

Section 1 A Review of Osteoporosis

Introduction

Osteoporosis may be defined as a reduction in bone mass per unit volume such that fractures may occur with minimal trauma. It is the most common metabolic bone disease in the Western world. There are many causes, but by far the most common and most important is postmenopausal osteoporosis. This affects most women by the end of their lives.

Despite an increasing awareness of the importance of osteoporosis in some sections of the population, many women are not aware of the condition, do not appreciate the way in which it may affect their lives and, most importantly, do not understand that it is preventable. It is the duty of healthcare professionals to provide women with an impartial account of the current knowledge regarding osteoporosis.

1 Epidemiology

Age- and gender-specific incidence and prevalence

Osteoporosis is the most important cause of fracture in the elderly in the Western world (Figure 1.1). In the USA, at least 1.3 million fractures per year are attributable to this condition[1]. Estimates of fracture frequency in the UK vary, but the combined annual incidence of fracture of the vertebrae, hip and distal forearm is approximately 200000, of which the majority are associated with osteoporosis. The cumulative lifetime risk of having an osteoporotic fracture is 2–4 times greater in women than in men[2]. It is difficult to calculate the economic cost of osteoporotic fractures, but it has been estimated that the annual cost of care for patients with proximal femoral fracture alone in the USA is $8 billion[3].

The three most common sites of osteoporotic fracture are the distal radius, the vertebral body and the upper femur. Fractures of the distal radius invariably result from a fall onto the outstretched hand. Each year, there are approximately 40000 such fractures in the UK[4] and 250000 in the USA[1]; in the UK, it has been estimated that 0.5% of women over the age of 70 years will sustain this fracture each year[5]. The rate of distal forearm fracture rises sharply after the age of 50 years in women, but changes little with age in men. After the age of 65 years, the rate in women does not appear to increase further.

In England in 1985, 37600 people aged 65 years and over sustained a fracture of the hip[6] and, in the USA in 1987, there were approximately 250000 hip fractures[1]. Although the increase in age-specific rate of hip fracture that occurred in the UK between the mid-1950s and 1980[7,8] appears to have ceased over the last 10 years[7], it is likely that the proportion of elderly women in the population will continue to increase. It has been estimated that a 15% increase may be anticipated in the rate of proximal femoral fractures during the next decade simply because of aging of the population[4]. The risk of hip fracture rises approximately 1.3% per annum in women aged over 65 years[9] and at half this rate in men[10]. At age 65 years, the incidence is 1–2 per thousand for women and 0.5–1 per thousand for men. By 85 years of age, the corresponding incidences in women and men are approximately 25 and 10 per thousand, respectively[10]. The present incidence suggests that 15% of women over age 65 years[11] and nearly a quarter of English women living to 90 years of age[6,12] can expect to have a hip fracture.

Hip fracture is an important cause of mortality and morbidity. Approximately 27% of women who sustain such a fracture die within a year[13]. Approximately half of the women who have had a hip fracture will experience long-term pain and disability[9], and 20% will have severely impaired mobility a year later[13]. In the USA, which does not have a domiciliary system such as has developed in the UK, half of the survivors of a fractured hip will enter long-term nursing-home care[14]. It has been recently estimated[15] that, within the next 10 years among white American women aged 45 years or more, there will be 5.2 million fractures of the hip, spine and forearm; 2 million person-years of fracture-related functional impairment; and $45.2 billion spent in direct medical costs.

There are few studies of the age-specific incidence of vertebral fracture as many fractures are subclinical. It has been estimated that only one-third of such events are brought to medical attention at the time of fracture[4]. The annual incidence in Rochester, Minnesota, is 0.5% at age 50 years, rising to 4% at age 85 years[14]. More data are available concerning prevalence in the apparently normal population. Smith and Risek[16] X-rayed 2063 women in Puerto Rico and southwestern Michigan, and found a prevalence of vertebral fracture that rose with age to a maximum of approximately 20% at around 70 years of age. More recent data[11] from 134 apparently normal women showed a prevalence of wedge fracture in approximately 60% of women over age 70 years and a prevalence of crushed vertebrae of 10%. Vertebral fractures are at least 10 times more common in women than in men[17].

A detailed and extensive study[18] of all fractures in the town of Malmö, Sweden, during the last 34 years has shown an increasing annual age-adjusted incidence of fracture of the hip, vertebrae and radius (Figure 1.2). This was attributed to reduced bone density resulting from declining physical activity, altered nutrition, and increased use of tobacco and/or alcohol[18].

Osteoporosis is an important cause of mortality and morbidity not only in the Western countries since the number of elderly women is increasing world-wide, most rapidly in Asia, Latin America, the Middle East and Africa. It has been estimated that these regions will account for more than 70% of the estimated 6.26 million fractures expected in the year 2050[3].

Relationship of bone density to fracture

Studies in which progressively increasing forces were applied to human femoral neck preparations *in vivo* have shown that the force necessary to cause fracture is linearly related to bone density[19,20]. There is little doubt that the risk of fracture is greatest in those women whose bone density is lowest.

Several prospective studies using modern methods of bone density measurement have shown a significant association between bone density and fracture risk in the female population. In the study of Hui and co-workers[21], single-photon absorptiometry (SPA) was used to measure bone density at the mid-radius in 521 white women who were followed up for an average of approximately 6.5 years. Fracture risk (excluding spinal fractures) increased with age and with decreasing radial bone density after age adjustment. The rate of increase in fracture risk with declining bone density appeared to be greater in the older age groups and in those with the lowest bone density. Overall, the risk of hip fracture alone increased 1.9 times with each g/cm decrease in radial bone mass (Figure 1.3).

Using SPA measurement at the distal and mid-radius, Gärdsell and colleagues[22] estimated bone density in 1076 women who were followed up for 11 years. The fracture risk was up to 7½ times greater in the 10% of women with the lowest bone densities compared with the 10% who had the highest densities. A larger study of 9704 white women used similar methods and followed up those women who had had bone density measured in the radius and os calcis. An increased risk of hip, humeral shaft and wrist fractures was found in those with the lowest bone densities[23,24].

Although there are correlations between bone density in the radius with those in the spine (Figure 1.4) and hip[25,26], the risk of hip fracture is more strongly associated with the bone density in the proximal femur than in the radius[27,28]. Similarly, vertebral bone density is likely to be the best predictor of spinal fracture[28–30]. The relationship between fracture risk and bone density measured directly at the hip and spine is stronger than that of bone density measured at peripheral sites[31].

Hip geometry may be an additional factor in fracture risk. A recent study[32] of hip axis length showed that this measurement was greater in women with osteoporotic fracture than in those without, suggesting that this may be a predictor of fracture independent of bone mineral density.

Several studies[28,33–35] have measured bone mineral density using dual-photon absorptiometry in the contralateral hip of women who had recently had a hip fracture and compared the results with age-matched controls. In all of these, and in the majority of similar but less well-conducted studies, the mean bone mineral density in women who had fractures was less than that in the controls. However, differences in the distributions of bone mineral density showed considerable overlap between the fracture and control groups. This has been interpreted by some authors to indicate that bone mineral density measurement at these sites is a poor predictor of fracture risk[12]. However, such a conclusion cannot be drawn from these data because the absence of fracture in women in the control group does not imply that they are not at risk of fracture in the future. Bone mineral density measurements are not intended to be a diagnostic test for fracture[36]. Serum cholesterol levels do not discriminate between subjects with or without coronary artery disease[37] but, as with bone mineral density measurements, can predict adverse health outcomes[38].

Relationship of falls to fracture

Although bone mineral density is closely associated with the risk of fracture, it does not account for all of the variation in fracture rate in the population. Age appears to be an important factor that is independent of bone mineral density. Thus, for any given bone mineral density, the fracture rate increases with age[21,39]. It is likely that the increased rate of falls known to occur with advancing age[40] is mainly responsible for this association. One report has shown that perimenopausal women fall more than age-matched men[41], and an increase in the rate of falls around the time of the menopause may be responsible for the sharp increase in the incidence of distal forearm fracture seen in women, but not men, at the age of 50 years[10]. Neuromuscular and visual impairment are predictors of hip fracture in elderly mobile women. A slower gait, poor heel-to-toe walking and reduced visual acuity have been reported to be independent predictors of hip fracture in a French study of 7575 women over 75 years of age[42].

It has been suggested that the relative roles of falls and reduced bone mineral density as contributors to the risk of fracture is different for the three most common osteoporotic fracture types[43]. Fractures of the distal radius may be more influenced by the rate of falls than low bone mineral density whereas the rate of fracture of the vertebral body, greatest in an older population, may be mainly related to low bone mineral density. The rate of distal forearm fracture does not appear to increase significantly in women over 65 years old whereas the rate of femoral neck fracture increases steadily with age as the rate of falls rises and bone mineral density declines. The vast majority of femoral fractures in the elderly are caused by simple falls on a level surface rather than more violent trauma[4]. It has been demonstrated that fractures of the femoral neck are more likely to occur in those who fall and have insufficient dexterity to use their hands to break their descent and thus fall directly onto their hip[44].

2 Bone structure

Cortical and trabecular bone

Bone provides the strength and rigidity of the skeleton as well as acting as a reservoir of calcium and other mineral salts. It is a highly vascular, mineralized connective tissue of cells in a fibrous organic matrix permeated by inorganic bone salts. The collagen framework varies from an almost random network to highly organized sheets or helical bundles of parallel fibers. Mature bone may be classified into two types, cortical or compact, and trabecular or cancellous.

Cortical bone is always found on the outside of bones and surrounds the trabecular bone (Figure 2.1). Approximately 80% of the skeleton is cortical bone. The architecture and amount of cortical bone at any site are related to its function at that area. Cortical bone is porous, but the ratio of solid tissue to space is considerably higher than for trabecular bone. Cortical bone is made up of a collection of cylindrical units termed Haversian systems, which run parallel to the outer surface of the bone. Each Haversian system has a central Haversian canal containing a neurovascular bundle, and each canal is surrounded by concentric lamellae of bony tissue (Figure 2.2). The lamellae are separated by small spaces termed lacunae, which are connected to each other and to the central Haversian canal by small channels called canaliculi. Osteocytes are found within the lacunae and extend cytoplasmic processes into the canaliculi. The gaps between the Haversian systems are made up of interstitial bone which consists of similar tissue elements, but in a less organized pattern. Haversian systems are separated from one another by cement lines which are strongly basophilic, have a high content of inorganic matrix, and correspond to areas of bone resorption and deposition.

Trabecular bone is found in the middle of bones such as the vertebrae, pelvis and other flat bones, and at the ends of the long bones. It consists mainly of more fragmented systems of Haversian lamellae and lacunae covered by numerous cement lines separated by large spaces filled with bone marrow. Trabecular bone receives its blood supply from the surrounding tissues. The high surface area-to-volume ratio of trabecular bone indicates that it is far more metabolically active compared with cortical bone and has the potential to change its density more rapidly.

Bone cells

There are three main types of bone cells: osteoblasts, osteoclasts and osteocytes.

Osteoblasts

These cells originate from bone marrow-derived stromal cells[45] and are responsible for the deposition of the extracellular matrix and its mineralization[46].

They are highly differentiated columnar-shaped cells (20–30 μm in diameter), usually found in a layer one-cell thick intimately apposed to areas of bone formation or remodeling (Figure 2.3). They have a cellular structure that includes extensive endoplasmic reticulum, a large Golgi complex and other cellular characteristics in keeping with their role as protein-synthesizing and -secreting cells. Whereas the 'plump' osteoblasts are active in bone formation (Figure 2.4), flatter and more inactive or 'resting' osteoblasts form the lining cells on the surface of bone. These lining cells may be responsible for removing the thin layer of osteoid which coats the bone surface, thus exposing the bone for osteoclastic resorption.

Osteoclasts

Osteoclasts are responsible for the resorption of calcified bone and cartilage (Figures 2.5 and 2.6). They are derived from hemopoietic stem cells and are formed by the fusion of mononuclear cell precursors[47]. Their morphological and phagocytic characteristics are similar to other cells of the mononuclear phagocytic cell line. They are typically large (up to 200 000 μm^3) and may contain up to 100 nuclei. The cells show cellular polarity, and resorption occurs along the 'ruffled' border of the cell apposed to the bone surface. The cytoplasm adjacent to this surface is devoid of organelles, but is rich in actin filaments and other microfilament-associated proteins[48], suggesting that this area contains the source of osteoclastic bone adhesion.

Osteocytes

Osteocytes are osteoblasts that remain behind in lacunae (Figure 2.7) when the bone-forming surface advances. They are the result of osteoblasts 'self-entombed' by their own bone matrix-secreting activity. As they become further isolated from the bone-forming surface, their protein synthesizing activity declines, the size of the endoplasmic reticulum and Golgi apparatus decreases, and the mitochondrial content falls. Osteocytes communicate with one another via cytoplasmic processes (Figure 2.8) that pass through the bone canaliculi. These processes may help to coordinate the response of bone to stress or deformation.

Bone proteins and minerals

Normal adult bone is termed lamellar bone. Each lamella is a thin plate 5–7 μm thick and made up of bone matrix consisting of protein fibers impregnated with bone salts. In each lamella, the protein fibers are largely orientated parallel to one another (Figure 2.9). The organic matrix constitutes 30–40%, and mineral salts 60–70%, of the dry weight of bone. Water makes up 20% of the weight of the matrix of mature bone.

The principal organic component in bone is type I collagen, which constitutes 90–95% of the organic matrix. It is a heteropolymer of two α1 chains and one α2 chain wound together in a triple helix. The important ionic components of the bone matrix are calcium, phosphate, magnesium, carbonate, hydroxyl, fluoride, citrate and chloride. The most important crystalline component of bone is hydroxyapatite [Ca10(PO4)6(OH)2], found as needle-shaped crystals 20–40 nm in length and 3–6 nm in breadth, generally lying with their long axes parallel to the collagen fibers. The other bone mineral ions are found in association with the surface of the hydroxyapatite crystals or they may replace phosphate ions within the crystals.

Bone remodeling

Bone is remodeled by osteoclasts and osteoblasts working in combination in a cycle of activity that lasts around 3–6 months. The resorption of bone by osteoclasts and its replacement by osteoblasts are normally 'coupled' together, which ensures that the processes of bone destruction and formation are more or less matched. This coupling is probably mediated by as yet unidentified cellular messengers produced by each cell type.

In the remodeling process (Figure 2.10), the osteoclast moves to an area of bone to be remodeled and secretes lactate or hydrogen ions through its ruffled cell border onto the bone surface to create an acid environment into which proteases such as proteoglycanase and collegenase are secreted from within the cell[49]. The bone matrix is then broken down by these enzymes, perhaps with the assistance of calcium chelating ions, such as citrate, which help to solubilize minerals (Figures 2.11 and 2.12). It is possible that released proteins such as bone morphogenic proteins act as signals or 'coupling factors' for the osteoblasts. After breakdown of the bone matrix is complete, the osteoclasts disappear. Several days later, osteoblasts move to the remodeling site, first to deposit extracellular matrix and, subsequently, to control its mineralization[46,50]. The chief protein secreted is type I collagen. The remodeling process occurs in both cortical (Figures 2.13 and 2.14) and trabecular (Figure 2.15) bone.

A recent study of osteoid seams, resorption cavities and bone structural units in iliac crest trabecular bone suggests that the above explanation of bone remodeling may be overly simplistic. It appears that, in some remodeling units, bone formation may start before complete resorption, bone resorption may be arrested in some cavities, and bone may be formed on quiescent bone surfaces[51]. The results of further studies are awaited.

Regulation of bone cell activity

Bone cell activity may be regulated by local or systemic factors (Table 2.1).

Table 2.1 Factors affecting bone resorption and formation (some assignments are tentative)

Factors	Resorption	Formation
Systemic		
PTH/PTH-related peptide	+	±
1,25-dihydroxyvitamin D_3	+	±
Calcitonin	–	?+
Estrogen, androgen	–	+
Glucocorticoid	+	±
Retinoid	±	±
Insulin	?	+
Growth hormone	?	+
Thyroid hormone	+	±
Local		
Prostanoid	±	+
Interleukin-1	+	±
Interleukin-4	–	?
Interleukin-6	?+	?
Colony-stimulating factor	+	–
Tumor necrosis factor	+	?
Interferon-γ	–	?
Leukemia inhibitory factor	+	?
Insulin-like growth factors I and II	?	+
Transforming growth factor-β	+	?
Epidermal growth factor	+	?
Transforming growth factor-α	±	+
Bone morphogenic protein	?	+
Platelet-derived growth factor	?	+
Fibroblast growth factor	?	?
Vasoactive intestinal peptide	+	?
Calcitonin gene-related peptide	–	?
Heparin	+	?
Miscellaneous		
Proton	+	?–
Calcium	–	+
Phosphate	+	?
Fluoride	–	+
Bisphosphonate	–	?
Antiestrogen	–	?+
Gallium nitrate	–	?
Alcohol, tobacco	?	–
Electric current	+	+
Immobilization, weightlessness	+	–
Stress, exercise	±	+

Systemic factors

The three main systemic hormones that regulate calcium homeostasis (calcitonin, vitamin D and parathyroid hormone) all appear to have direct effects on bone cells. The principal action of calcitonin is to inhibit bone resorption. Parathyroid hormone produces changes in the shape of osteoblasts which is thought to be indicative of increased bone resorption[52] (Figure 2.16). It is probable that 1,25-dihydroxyvitamin D_3 has effects on both osteoblasts and osteoclasts. It increases osteoblastic production of osteocalcin and alkaline phosphatase, and stimulates osteoclastic differentiation and multinucleation[53].

Estrogen has an important action in preserving bone, and estrogen hormone replacement therapy (HRT) is the most commonly used treatment for preventing osteoporosis. The mechanism of action is not known, but direct actions on bone cells have been suggested. Functional estradiol receptors[54,55] and estrogen receptor-related protein[56] have been identified in osteoblast-like cells (Figure 2.17), albeit at very low levels[57], but not in osteoclasts (Figure 2.18). It has been proposed that estrogens may block the actions of various cytokines that promote the transformation of progenitor cells into osteoclasts[58]. Several studies have shown that estrogens increase calcitonin secretion in both pre- and post-menopausal women[59-62], although some studies have not[63]. Calcitonin secretion has been shown to be reduced in studies of established osteoporotics compared with controls[26,64], but other studies have not shown this effect[65]. It is possible that the different results of calcitonin studies are due to variations in the ability of different antisera to recognize different heterogeneous molecular species or because of differences in extraction techniques.

Local factors

Local factors include cytokines, growth factors, other peptides and nitric oxide. A cytokine is a peptide produced by a cell that acts as an autocrine, paracrine or endocrine mediator[53]. A large and increasing number of cytokines have been shown to have an effect on bone. It is presently thought that the most important are interleukin-1 (IL-1), interleukin-6 (IL-6), tumor necrosis factor (TNF) and interferon (IFN)-γ[63].

IL-1 is a monocyte/macrophage product found in two forms, α and β, which appear to have similar biological activity. IL-1 stimulates some osteoblast-like cells to secrete proteinases, such as collagenase and stromelysin, which may contribute to the breakdown of connective tissue matrices[58]. The production of IL-1 after the menopause is increased and, in patients with osteoporosis, may be suppressed by estrogen therapy[66]. A recent report has demonstrated that IL-1α, IL-1β and IL-1β mRNA are expressed significantly more in bone from osteoporotic women than from women with normal bone mineral density or postmenopausal women taking HRT[67].

TNF is also found in α and β forms which are similar in activity to each other and to IL-1. Studies *in vitro* show that both TNF and IL-1 inhibit bone resorption and formation[68,69]. IL-1 and TNF may act in synergy and induce the production of each other as well as other cytokines. Production of TNF may be markedly inhibited by estrogen treatment in postmenopausal women, but not in premenopausal women or men[58].

IFN-γ inhibits IL-1- or TNF-induced bone resorption, but has less effect on resorption stimulated by parathyroid hormone or 1,25-dihydroxyvitamin D_3[70] and may be considered a potential antagonist to IL-1 and TNF.

Numerous growth factors that directly influence bone cell activity have been identified and include platelet-derived growth factor (PDGF), insulin-like growth factors and transforming growth factor (TGF)-β. PDGF stimulates bone resorption, is mitogenic for fibroblasts and may mediate the mitogenic effects of IL-1[71]. TGF-β is produced in an inactive form which is activated by an acid environment. It has been postulated that TGF-β may be released from bone matrix during absorption, and affect osteoblastic and osteoclastic activity[58], and may have a role in the regulation of osteoclast progenitors in the bone marrow[72]. Estrogens may prevent bone loss by limiting osteoclastic lifespan through promotion of apoptosis mediated by TGF-β[73].

Of the other peptides involved in the regulation of bone cell activity, prostaglandins may be the most important. Their actions on bone have been extensively studied *in vitro*, but their physiological role is still uncertain[74]. The ability of IL-1, TNF and TGF-β to stimulate bone resorption may be partly mediated by increased prostaglandin synthesis[75], and production of these cytokines may be influenced by prostaglandins. It has been suggested that low concentrations of prostanoids may alter osteoclast mobility[58]. The bone-preserving effect of estrogen in osteoporotic women may be partly due to an action in influencing prostaglandin E_2 production in bone[76].

Nitric oxide (NO) has recently been found to have important effects on bone. Forms of nitric oxide synthase are expressed by bone-derived cells, and IL-1, TNF and IFN-γ are potent stimulators of nitric oxide production[77]. When combined with other cytokines, IFN-γ induces nitric oxide production, which suppresses osteoclast formation and activity of mature osteoclasts. High nitric oxide concentrations inhibit cells of the osteoblast lineage and nitric oxide production may be partly responsible for the inhibitory effects of cytokines on osteoblast proliferation. At lower nitric oxide concentrations, the effects appear to be different. Moderate induction of nitric oxide potentiates bone resorption and promotes osteoblast-like cell proliferation and function[78]. It is likely that nitric oxide is one of the molecules produced by osteoblasts that regulate osteoclast activity[79,80].

Proton secretion by the ruffled border of osteoclasts is necessary to solubilize bone mineral and degrade the organic matrix of bone. One or two protons are secreted for every Ca^{++} liberated[81]. This secretion is mediated via an electrogenic H(+)-adenosine-triphosphatase (ATPase) coupled to a chloride channel in the ruffled membrane. Antiresorptive agents such as tiludronate may partially act by inhibiting H(+)-ATPase[82]. Changes in pH may be of importance as the regulation of bone resorption and osteoclasts is acutely sensitive to pH.

Many other systemic and local factors have been shown to act directly on bone cells. For a full description, the interested reader is referred to other texts[53,58,83].

3 Pathogenesis

The major factors that determine whether a person develops osteoporosis are the maximum (peak) bone density that is achieved and the amount that is subsequently lost. Bone quality and architecture may also be important.

Peak bone mass

Peak bone mass in men and women is probably achieved soon after their skeletal growth ceases[84,85] (Figures 3.1 and 3.2). The bone mass at skeletal maturity differs between the sexes, being 30–50% greater in men than in women[86,87]. However, the lean/bone mass ratios in mature men and women are similar[68], suggesting that both sexes at that time have an equal capacity to withstand mechanical trauma.

Peak bone mass is largely determined by genetic factors. The variance in bone mineral density between dizygotic twins is much greater than in monozygotic twins[88], and the daughters of women who have had a hip fracture have lower than average bone mineral density[89]. Genetic factors are almost certainly the reason for racial differences in bone mineral density, with a higher bone mineral density in blacks compared with whites[90] and no evidence of a change in the incidence of osteoporosis in people who migrate from an area of low incidence to one of high incidence.

Environmental influences on peak bone mass include diet and exercise. Some studies suggest that calcium intake during childhood and adolescence influences peak bone mass[91–93], but there is little evidence that calcium supplementation in school-age children has any effect[74]. It is possible that general dietary intake in early life is as important as calcium intake as a determinant of peak bone mass[94].

Although it is well established that long-term physical exercise results in regional increases in bone mass[95] (Figure 3.3) and immobilization leads to bone loss, it is uncertain whether a lifetime of activity reduces the risk of hip fracture[95,96]. Surprisingly few studies have examined the effect of exercise in early adult life on peak bone mass. A preliminary study by Kanders and colleagues[91] suggests that both an adequate intake of calcium and an active lifestyle are both necessary for maximizing bone mineral density in early adult life. It has been postulated that exercise is the prime environmental influence on peak bone mass, which is greater in the presence of adequate calcium intake[17]. Data from a recent UK study suggest that, after allowing for body build, physical activity is the major determinant of peak bone density[97].

Excessive exercise may lead to hypothalamic-induced hypoestrogenism which, in turn, results in reduced bone mineral density[98–100]. Thus, physical activity cannot counteract the effects of hormone deprivation on the skeleton. Prolonged periods of hypoestrogenism during young adult life, such as are seen in anorexia nervosa, reduce peak bone density and predispose to osteoporosis.

Smoking, alcohol and lifestyle factors

Smoking is associated with a reduced peak bone mass[85,101], earlier menopause[102] and thinness[103], all of which are risk factors for osteoporotic fracture. It appears to reduce bone mineral density by a mechanism that is independent of its effect on weight or estrogen metabolism[101]. Data from a recent twin study suggest that women who smoke 20 cigarettes a day throughout adulthood will, by the time of the menopause, have an average bone mineral density deficit of 5–10% compared with non-smokers[104].

It is not known whether the lower bone mineral density found in alcoholics[105] is mainly due to inadequate dietary intake, poor exercise or a direct effect of alcohol in reducing osteoblastic activity[106], but it is likely to be a combination of these factors. Although the bone mineral density in the proximal femur has been shown to be significantly lower in premenopausal women who consume more than two drinks per day compared with those who consume less[85], the differences are small. A recent Finnish study of risk factors for fracture in 3140 women followed up for a mean of 2.4 years showed greater alcohol intake in those who developed fracture than those who did not[107]. This finding may be due to an effect of alcohol on balance rather than bone mineral density.

Increased parity is associated with increased bone mineral density. A recent retrospective UK study[108] of 825 women found a 1% gain in bone mineral density per live births that was independent of other risk factors.

Bone loss

Although one study[28] has suggested that integral spinal bone mineral density declines linearly throughout life and another[109] found that at least 50% of trabecular bone in women is lost before the menopause, most authorities agree that the bone mineral density declines slowly in women until just before the menopause and that the loss increases considerably thereafter[85] (see Figures 3.1 and 3.2). Bone loss probably begins in the third or fourth decade of life and may be due, at least in men, to a decline in osteoblast function[110]. The decline in bone mineral density is around 0.5% per year.

In women, the bone mineral density appears to fall exponentially, commencing just before the menopause[111,112] when ovarian function begins to decline. This loss is chiefly due to the increased resorption of bone[113–116] superimposed on the effects of aging. The loss of bone is greatest initially and may be as much as 5% per year for vertebral trabecular bone[117,118]. The loss is even greater after oophorectomy[119]. The loss of cortical bone in the perimenopausal years is slower than for trabecular bone[117,120–122] and, after 8–10 years, the rate of total bone loss declines to less than 1% per annum.

There is accumulating evidence that the rate of perimenopausal bone loss varies considerably between women. Approximately 35% of women lose large amounts of bone mineral at the menopause; they are the 'fast' bone losers. A fast rate of bone loss and a low bone mineral density may contribute equally to future risk of fracture[123]. Fast bone losers may lose approximately 50% more bone mass at the wrist, spine and hip within 12 years of menopause than slow bone losers[124]. Some reports suggest that this difference is not related to initial bone mineral content, parity or smoking habits, but to estrogen levels and fat mass[125]. Fat postmenopausal women have higher endogenous estrogen production[126,127] and it appears that fast bone losers have lower serum concentrations of estrogens than slow bone losers[128–130]. Some authors have demonstrated that perimenopausal white women with the highest bone masses lose most bone, in absolute terms, following the loss of ovarian function[118,119]. However, a recent prospective UK follow-up study of postmenopausal women over 5 years found no correlation between rate of bone loss in the forearm and spine and baseline bone density[131].

Bone architecture and quality

The structural architecture of bone has received little attention until recently. Recent research has focused upon trabecular bone loss and its response to treatment, as it is this bone type that shows the greatest metabolic activity (Figures 3.4–3.7). Trabecular bone loss may result from thinning or loss of trabeculae. The latter leads to a reduction in 'connectedness' of the bone elements (Figures 3.8 and 3.9), which may then have no functional value, but will contribute to the bone mineral density.

However, there is evidence that a reduced connectedness is also associated with a greater reduction in bone mineral density than is trabecular thinning[132]. Both processes appear to occur with advancing age in both sexes, but disconnectedness is found more often in women[133]. Some data suggest that trabecular thinning is due to reduced bone formation whereas erosion is secondary to increased bone turnover, which occurs during the perimenopausal years[134]. Increased bone turnover by itself will increase fracture risk because of an increased likelihood of trabecular perforation. Conversely, therapeutic reductions in bone turnover may reduce fracture risk even before significant increases in density have been achieved.

New techniques of computed analysis of the structure of iliac crest bone biopsies have made possible the measurement of indices of bone architecture such as trabecular pattern, trabecular separation and number[135]. Such techniques may enable more detailed study of the effects of menopause and its treatment on bone architecture.

4 Biochemical changes

Calcium, vitamin D and parathyroid hormone

In the normal person whose bone mass is being maintained, approximately 6 mmol of calcium enters and leaves the skeleton each day[136], and the amount of calcium leaving the body in the urine and digestive juices is matched by the amount absorbed from the gut. Plasma calcium is chiefly regulated by the actions of parathyroid hormone, and vitamin D and its derivatives on the kidney, skeleton and gut.

Parathyroid hormone secretion increases in response to a fall in plasma calcium and acts directly on the kidney to increase tubular calcium reabsorption. It increases renal synthesis of 1,25-dihydroxyvitamin D which then acts on the gut to increase the active transport of calcium. Increasing parathyroid hormone levels result in increased bone turnover, with resorption predominating when parathyroid hormone levels become supraphysiological. An increase in serum calcium reduces parathyroid hormone secretion and stimulates the release of calcitonin.

Calcium metabolism changes considerably around the time of the menopause. Both bone resorption and formation increase, but with formation less so than resorption, leading to a negative calcium balance of approximately 50 mg/day. This calcium is excreted in the urine. The plasma calcium rises at the menopause[137], leading to a small homeostatic decline in levels of both parathyroid hormone and 1,25-dihydroxyvitamin D in early postmenopausal women[138]. The lower level of 1,25-dihydroxyvitamin D, in turn, results in a fall in intestinal calcium absorption[139]. Compared with normal subjects, osteoporotic women show differences in calcium balance, plasma calcium and calcium-regulating hormones similar to those between pre- and post-menopausal women[26,140]. This suggests that neither a primary defect in calcium absorption[141] nor renal endocrine failure[142] is the cause of osteoporosis in the majority of cases.

Urinary calcium excretion

The early morning urinary fasting calcium-to-creatinine ratio may reflect the difference between bone resorption and formation, as the influence of intestinal calcium absorption is minimal. Fasting urinary calcium-to-creatinine ratios increase after the menopause and fall in response to antiresorption therapy.

Biochemical markers of bone formation

Alkaline phosphatase

The principal role of alkaline phosphatase is probably to hydrolyze pyrophosphate and therefore permit growth of hydroxyapatite crystals on newly synthesized mineralizing osteoid[143]. Levels of serum alkaline phosphatase are raised by increased bone turnover due to increased osteoblastic production (Figure 4.1) but, as there are many non-bony causes of elevated serum alkaline phosphatase levels, interpretation is difficult. Assays of bone-specific alkaline phosphatase have been developed using chemical inhibition[144], gel electrophoresis[145] and heat inactivation[146]. The generation of specific monoclonal antibodies to bone isoenzymes should lead to even more sensitive tests in the future[147].

Procollagen extension peptides

During the formation of collagen from procollagen, N- and C-terminal peptides are released. A molecule incorporating three C-terminal fragments (PColl-1-C) may be measured in plasma, and appears to be raised in Paget's disease and reduced in this disease with successful treatment using calcitonin or bisphosphonate[113]. In a recent study[148], circulating levels of these fragments were lowered by estrogen and progestogen HRT in 12 osteoporotic patients. These fragments may prove to be valuable markers of bone formation.

Gla protein

Bone Gla protein (osteocalcin) is a non-collagenous protein synthesized exclusively by osteoblasts. It is a sensitive and specific marker of osteoblastic activity in a variety of metabolic bone diseases, including osteoporosis[128,149-151].

Biochemical markers of bone resorption

Urinary hydroxyproline

Hydroxyproline is a product of collagen breakdown and approximately 10% of the total production is excreted into the urine as the peptide-bound form. Collection of urine for measurement of total 24-h urinary hydroxyproline is inconvenient for patients and has, to a large extent, been replaced by the fasting urinary hydroxyproline-to-creatinine ratio, which may be determined from a small urine sample. Urinary hydroxyproline may be increased by meat and fish in the diet, acute infections and collagen turnover in other tissues such as skin and cartilage; thus, unless these factors have been eliminated, results should be viewed with caution[143].

Pyridinoline cross-links

Lysyl pyridinoline cross-links appear to be specific to mature type I bone collagen and are measurable in urine because of their natural fluorescence. Urinary pyridinoline and deoxypyridinoline concentrations are directly related to bone-matrix degradation. These markers are found to be elevated in postmenopausal normal and osteoporotic women compared with premenopausal women, and reduced with estrogen replacement therapy[152,153]. Urinary pyridinoline cross-link excretion has been reported to be superior to urinary hydroxyproline in discriminating between women with or without osteoporosis[154]. Serum levels of these markers also appear to reflect bone formation and resorption rates[155].

Type I collagen telopeptides

Carboxy-terminal telopeptides of type I collagen may be measured in serum and appear to discriminate between osteoporotic and non-osteoporotic women[156,157]. However, as markers of resorption, they may not be sufficiently sensitive to detect the changes induced by HRT[158].

Peripheral serum levels of IL-1 and IL-6 have, so far, not been found to be useful markers of osteoporosis[159]. Attempts to combine markers of bone turnover to improve sensitivity and specificity of detection of low bone mineral density have proved disappointing[160].

5 Diagnosis

Radiography

Radiography reveals recognizable bone loss only when 25–30% of bone density has been lost, at which time osteoporosis is generally considered to have developed. In the past, radiogrammetry has been used to assess bone mineral density of the peripheral skeleton, usually at the metacarpals. The metacarpal cortical thickness was used for many years to diagnose and predict the risk of osteoporosis. However, the sensitivity of radiography is poor[161,162], and the results of metacarpal measurement do not reflect bone mineral density at more important sites such as the hip and spine[121,163]. Although there is a correlation between bone mineral density in the peripheral and central skeleton[25,121] (see Figure 1.6), the association is not strong enough to predict central bone mineral density from peripheral measurements in a given subject[121,164]. At present, the main role of radiography is in the diagnosis of fractures secondary to osteoporosis (Figures 5.1–5.6).

Single-photon and single X-ray absorptiometry

Single-photon absorptiometry (SPA; Figure 5.7) involves passing a collimated beam of monoenergetic photons from a radioiodine (^{125}I) source through a limb and measuring the transmitted radiation, using a sodium iodide scintillation detector. However, SPA has now been largely superseded by single X-ray absorptiometry (SXA). The dose of radiation with both methods is low. There is differential absorption of photons by bone and soft tissues which allows the total bone mineral content in the path of the beam to be calculated and expressed in grams per centimeter. The method cannot differentiate between cortical and trabecular bone, and interference from surrounding tissue limits its use to measurement of peripheral sites, such as the distal or mid-radius. At the mid-radius, the cortical-to-trabecular bone ratio is approximately 95:5 whereas, at the distal radius, it is about 75:25[15]. Measurements from the latter bone are thus more likely to reflect more metabolically active trabecular bone mineral density (Figure 5.8). The precision error (reproducibility of the result on repeat testing of the same subject at the same site) for SXA is about 0.3% at either site[165]. Both SPA and SXA are well tolerated by patients and require little time. However, their main drawback is their inability to measure bone mineral density at the hip or spine.

Dual-photon absorptiometry and dual-energy X-ray absorptiometry

Dual-photon absorptiometry (DPA) uses ^{153}Gd (gadolinium) as a source and measures bone mineral density by determining the absorption of two beams of photons at two different energies (Figure 5.9); however, this method has now been superseded by dual-energy X-ray absorptiometry (DEXA; Figure 5.10). Both methods are able to measure bone mineral density (as mass/area) in the proximal femur and lumbar spine as well as the total body, but they cannot differentiate between cortical and trabecular bone. The cortical-to-trabecular ratio is 1:2 in the spine[166] and 3:1 in the femoral neck[17]. Thus, measurements of the total BMD at these sites are more a reflection of trabecular bone density than are measurements taken in the peripheral skeleton.

DEXA is similar to DPA except that the radioisotope source is replaced by an X-ray source. This enables bone mineral density to be measured at the hip or spine with greater precision than with the methods described above (precision error: 0.5–2%). The technique is able to measure bone mineral density in the spine (Figures 5.10–5.13), proximal femur (Figures 5.14 and 5.15) and the total body (Figures 5.16 and 5.17). The X-ray source produces a higher photon flux than either ^{125}I or ^{153}Gd so that the scanning time is shorter (around 5min at each site). The radiation dose is also less, approximately 1mrem for each site. Most techniques involve measurements taken from a posteroanterior view. Recent reports suggest that lateral views may be better than posteroanterior views in the diagnosis of osteoporosis[167], and that volumetric bone mineral density measured by DEXA from both posteroanterior and lateral views may better predict fracture than DEXA and posteroanterior view alone[168]. This has not become generally accepted.

Quantitative computed tomography

Quantitative computed tomography (CT; Figure 5.18) with a suitable software package enables the absorption by different calcified tissues to be determined so that areas of particular interest, such as the vertebral body (which has a cortical-to-trabecular ratio of approximately 5:95) may be studied[166]. The technique measures true density[119,166,169] with the results expressed in g/cm^3. Tissue density is compared with a calibration phantom (Figures 5.19 and 5.20). New developments include software automation for determining the region of interest and the use of solid calibration phantoms (Figures 5.21 and 5.22).

At present, CT scanning is chiefly used to assess trabecular bone density in the spine although, recently, it has been reported to be useful in measuring radial density[170]. The precision and accuracy of spinal measurements are approximately 2–4% and 5–10%, respectively, but there is considerable variation depending on the method used.

Dual-energy scanning (with double the radiation dose) may improve the accuracy, but worsen the precision. The radiation dose (200mrem per single-energy vertebral body scan[171]) and cost are considerably greater than with the methods described above.

An advantage of CT is that trabecular bone is distinguished from cortical bone (Figure 5.23), and extraosseous calcium, which artificially increases the bone density measured by DEXA, is readily identified (Figures 5.24 and 5.25)[172]. Trabecular diameter and intertrabecular spaces can be measured using high-resolution CT, and abnormal trabecular architecture can be identified[173]. Future developments, in particular, three-dimensional CT (Figures 5.26 and 27), will vastly improve the quality of the image and may prove suitable for quantitation.

Nuclear magnetic resonance scanning

Preliminary reports of magnetic resonance imaging of the radius indicate that density measurements correlate well with trabecular bone mineral density as measured by CT[169], and that imaging of the spine using nuclear magnetic resonance can distinguish osteoporotics and non-osteoporotics[174]. Different nuclear magnetic resonance imaging techniques are currently under investigation[169,175].

Neutron activation analysis

In vivo neutron activation analysis (IVNAA) measures total body calcium by irradiating the body with thermal neutrons and examining the ^{49}Ca part of the gamma ray spectrum that results[176] (Figure 5.28). The availability of this method is limited, and few long-term controlled studies of its use in patients receiving treatment for osteoporosis have been published. The accuracy error for total body calcium is 3–5% and the precision error is 8–10%[176]. The total body irradiation time is approximately 60 s followed by 20 min in a whole-body radioactivity monitor. The radiation received during total body IVNAA is 1 rem, which is approximately 1000 times that with total skeletal assessment using DEXA. Measurement of specific bony areas of interest is not possible and this, coupled with the high radiation dose involved, renders IVNAA of limited use at present in the diagnosis or study of osteoporosis.

Ultrasonography

The attenuation of ultrasound signals during their passage through bone may be measured by determining the reduction in ultrasound signal amplitude. Broadband ultrasonic attenuation describes the increase in ultrasound attenuation over a partic- ular frequency range, typically 0.2–0.6 MHz, and may be used to estimate bone mineral density of the calcaneus (Figure 5.29)[177]. The heel is placed in a small water bath between two ultrasonic transducers at a fixed separation. One transducer acts as a transmitter, the other as a receiver. The measurement takes between 1 and 10 min, depending on the type of machinery, and involves no ionizing radiation. The velocity of ultrasound through the heel can also be measured[178].

Several studies have shown significant correlations between calcaneus broadband ultrasonic attenuation and spine or hip bone mineral density as measured by DEXA[179] and DPA[180–182], although a recent report found a poor relationship between broadband ultrasonic attenuation and DEXA measurements of the spine and hip[183]. Wasnich and colleagues[184] reported that calcaneus bone mineral density (measured by SPA) was as effective as lumbar spine or radius bone mineral density in predicting fracture. A recent study[185] of 4698 women aged 69 years or more reported that the broadband ultrasonic attenuation at the calcaneus is related to the incidence of past fracture of the hip and that this relationship is partly independent of bone mineral density. Using a combination of both bone mineral density and broadband ultrasonic attenuation measurements may prove to have higher sensitivity and specificity for predicting fracture risk than the use of each method alone.

6 Treatment

The methods of drug treatment of osteoporosis may be broadly divided into those that retard bone resorption, such as estrogens, calcitonin and bisphosphonates, and those that stimulate bone formation, such as anabolic steroids and fluoride. Recently, combined regimens have been under investigation. Increasing the amount of exercise and eliminating the risk factors for falls have a part to play in the prevention of osteoporotic fractures.

Hormone replacement therapy

Estrogen therapy is the most commonly used prophylactic measure and has been shown to reduce the frequency of osteoporotic fracture. Until recently, few prospective studies of the effect of HRT on fracture risk had been published. In a recent report of 3140 peri- and postmenopausal women followed for a mean of 2.5 years, the age-adjusted risk of fracture was 0.75 (95% CI 0.5–0.96) for HRT users compared with non-users[186]. Several retrospective studies have shown that the use of estrogens for 5 years is associated with a 50% reduction in the risk of hip fracture[187–189] and a reduced rate of vertebral fracture[190]. Estrogens may reduce the rate of fracture by increasing mobility and dexterity, but the majority of their effect is likely to be due to their action on bone density.

Satisfactory prospective controlled studies of the effects of estrogen on bone density are also scarce. The study by Lindsay and colleagues[9] measured metacarpal density, using SPA, in 120 postmenopausal women who were randomized to one of four groups taking different dosages of conjugated equine estrogen and a control group. There was no reduction in mean bone density in women taking 0.625 mg/day and 1.25 mg/day over 2 years, but there was a mean fall in density of 5% and 8% in the two groups of women taking 0.3 mg/day and 0.15 mg/day, respectively, and a fall of 8% in the controls. Christiansen and co-workers[191] used SPA to examine the changes in forearm bone density over 1 year in 69 early postmenopausal women randomized to three different dosages of oral estradiol and a control group. Bone density in the control group fell by 2%, but rose by 1.5% and 0.8% in those women taking 4 mg/day and 2 mg/day of estradiol, respectively, and did not change in those taking 1 mg/day.

Munk-Jensen and colleagues[192] conducted a double-blind, randomized, placebo-controlled study of the effects of an oral continuous estrogen/progestogen HRT regimen and an oral sequential HRT regimen (with progestogen added for 10 of every 28 days) on 100 women who were within 2 years of the menopause. Spinal bone mineral content was measured by DPA, and forearm mineral content by SPA, for 1 year. The bone mineral content rose in all treated groups and fell in the controls. The rise in spine bone mineral contents for continuous estrogen/progestogen treatment (4.9%) was more than for sequential therapy (3.9%), but did not reach statistical significance.

Estradiol implants appear to preserve bone density. McKay Hart and colleagues[193] followed up 19 oophorectomized women treated with 50-mg estradiol implants every 6 months for 2 years. The bone mineral density in the lumbar spine (measured by DPA) increased by 4.3% per year. A similar increase of 3.3% per year in trabecular bone density (measured by CT) has been reported over a 3-year period with the same treatment regimen[194]. The results of a cross-sectional study comparing the effects of oral estrogens and implant estrogen and testosterone therapy on spine and femoral bone density suggested a greater rise in bone mineral density in women treated with implants[195]. The bone mineral density increases with implant therapy appear to be highest in women who have the highest estradiol levels during treatment[196].

Transdermal estrogen therapy appears to produce similar effects to oral therapy. Riis and co-workers[197] found increases in bone mineral density in the spine in postmenopausal women treated with percutaneous estrogen combined with oral progesterone. In a study of spine and hip bone density (using DPA) in 66 postmenopausal women randomized to receive either transdermal HRT (estradiol-17β at 0.05 mg daily with norethindrone acetate at 0.25 mg daily for 14 of every 28 days) or oral therapy (continuous equine estrogen at 0.625 mg daily with dl-norgestrel at 0.15 mg daily for 12 of every 28 days), and compared with a reference group studied concurrently[198], bone mineral density was measured at 6-month intervals for 3 years and skeletal turnover was assessed by serum measurements of calcium, phosphate and alkaline phosphatase, and by urine estimations of hydroxyproline/creatinine and calcium/creatinine excretion. Vertebral and femoral bone mineral density rose significantly in both treatment groups and fell in the reference group. The biochemical measurements indicated a significant reduction in bone turnover in the treated groups (Figures 6.1 and 6.2).

Several studies suggest that a small proportion of women taking estrogen at currently accepted 'bone-preserving' doses will not maintain their bone mineral density. This may be due to variations in the absorption of estrogen, failure of compliance or individual differences in the response of bone to estrogen. Unfortunately, the literature so far does not allow any firm conclusions to be drawn, as the designs of many of the studies showing loss of bone mineral density with standard doses of estrogen do not include sufficient data on compliance or estrogen levels[117,190]. Of the women treated with 0.05 mg/day of transdermal estrogen, 12% have been shown to lose forearm bone density[197]. Spinal bone density was not maintained in one-third of oophorectomized women treated with 0.625 mg/day of conjugated equine estrogen[190] and in 22% of women following a natural menopause[117]. It has been demonstrated that 12% of women taking either estradiol-17β at 0.05 mg/day with norethindrone acetate 0.25 mg/ day for 14 of every 28 days or continuous equine oestrogen at 0.625 mg/day with dl-norgestrel at 0.15 mg/day for 12 of every 28 days with good compliance for 3 years will show significant loss of bone in the proximal femur[198].

Withdrawal of estrogen treatment appears to result in bone loss at a rate similar to that in the immediate postmenopausal period[120,199]; thus, it is likely that the effect of estrogen on bone mineral density is to 'buy time'[200]. In women who discontinue treatment, the amount of bone 'bought' is probably the duration of estrogen use multiplied by the rate of bone loss during the slow phase (approximately 1% per year) after the period of fast loss in the early postmenopausal years (Figure 6.3).

Estrogen therapy may be most effective in elderly women. A recent report found that estrogen was most effective in preventing hip fractures in women over 75 years of age[201]. It has been suggested that an effective strategy to prevent fracture in postmenopausal women would be to target elderly women with a high risk of osteoporotic fracture in whom short periods of treatment appear to have profound effects on fracture risk[202].

The mechanism of effect of estrogens on bone is uncertain. Estrogens may have a direct effect on osteoblasts or on the cytokines that regulate osteoblast formation such as IL-1 or TNF[203]. They may also have an indirect effect on bone by increasing calcitonin secretion or by influencing local factors. Recent information suggests that, although HRT increases bone mineral density, it may not have an effect on trabecular architecture and is unable to reverse structural disruption in women with postmenopausal osteoporosis[204].

Selective estrogen receptor modulators

Concerns regarding the long-term effects of estrogen on the risk of breast cancer and on the endometrium have led to the development of selective estrogen receptor modulators (SERMS). Raloxifene is a non-steroidal benzothiophene that inhibits bone mineral density loss, but does not stimulate the endometrium. It does not appear to be a useful treatment for climacteric hot flushes.

In a 2-year multicenter, placebo-controlled, double-blind study, Delmas and co-workers[205] randomized 661 postmenopausal women to receive 30, 60 or 150 mg of raloxifene per day or placebo. Of these women, 55% had low bone mineral density. The densities of the hip and spine were measured by DEXA every 6 months. Biochemical markers of bone turnover were measured every 3 months and included serum osteocalcin, serum bone-specific alkaline phosphatase and the urinary type I collagen C-telopeptide-to-creatinine ratio. By the end of the study, 25% of the participants had dropped out.

Bone mineral density increased significantly in the lumbar spine, total hip, femoral neck and total body in all three treatment groups, and fell in the placebo group (Figures 6.4 and 6.5). The increase in bone mineral density at most sites was greatest in the group that received raloxifene 150 mg/day although, in the total hip, the greatest increase was seen in the 60 mg/day group. Compared with placebo, each of the treatments statistically signifi-

cantly decreased concentrations of the three markers of bone turnover (Figure 6.6).

A recent preliminary report[206] suggests that raloxifene may reduce the vertebral fracture risk in postmenopausal women with osteoporosis. In another multicenter 2-year study, 7705 women were randomized to receive placebo or raloxifene 60 mg/day or 120 mg/day. One or more incidences of vertebral fracture occurred in 5.5% of women; compared with those in the placebo group, women taking raloxifene had a relative risk of fracture of 0.56 (95% CI 0.46–0.68). A similar reduction in risk (RR 0.39; 95% CI 0.25–0.60) was observed in the 1% of women who had multiple incidences of vertebral fracture. Raloxifene and other SERMS may prove to be of value in the long-term prevention or treatment of osteoporosis.

Calcitonin

Calcitonin directly suppresses the activity of osteoclasts and also inhibits their recruitment (Figure 6.7). It has been isolated from a large number of animal species. Calcitonin from fish is the most resistant to degradation in humans and, thus, has the greatest potency per unit weight. It is not yet known whether calcitonins from other species will be more effective. Daily intramuscular salmon calcitonin at a relatively high dosage (100 IU) has been shown to prevent bone loss and slightly increase skeletal mass in women with osteoporotic fractures[207]. In healthy women, a much lower dose (20 IU) of synthetic human calcitonin, given subcutaneously three times a week in the early postmenopausal period, was as effective as estrogen in preventing spinal trabecular bone loss[208]. The inconvenience of injectable calcitonin has led to the development of alternative methods of administration. Reports of the use of salmon calcitonin suppositories have failed to show effects on spinal or femoral bone mineral density, or on markers of bone turnover[209], and the suppositories are reported to have poor tolerability[210]. However, studies of intranasal salmon calcitonin suggest that it may be of value in both the prevention and treatment of osteoporosis[211–216].

In a recent double-blind, placebo-controlled trial[217], the effects of intranasal salmon calcitonin on bone mineral density (as measured by DPA) were studied for 2 years in 117 postmenopausal women with reduced bone density. The subjects were randomized to receive salmon calcitonin 200 IU daily or three times a week, or placebo. Compared with placebo, daily salmon calcitonin resulted in no significant loss in lumbar bone mineral density over 2 years (Figure 6.8). In this group of women, those who were more than 5 years past the menopause showed the greatest response. Although there was no difference in changes in proximal femoral bone density among the three groups, bone mineral density did not fall significantly in women taking daily salmon calcitonin. Significant bone loss in both the spine and proximal femur was seen in women receiving thrice-weekly salmon calcitonin or placebo. There were no significant treatment-related adverse effects and salmon calcitonin was well tolerated.

More recently, the final results of a 5-year, double-blind, randomized, placebo-controlled study of the effects of calcitonin nasal spray (Miacalcic®/ Miacalcin® Nasal Spray) on vertebral fracture in postmenopausal women have been published in abstract[218]. A total of 1255 women with established osteoporosis were randomized to placebo, 100, 200 or 400 IU/day of nasal spray. All women were also given 1 g calcium and 400 IU vitamin D. A 36% reduction in risk of new vertebral fracture was observed in women taking 200 IU/day (relative risk = 0.64, 95% CI 0.47–0.97, p = 0.03). It appears that intranasal salmon calcitonin 200 IU daily is effective and safe for the prevention of bone loss in post-menopausal women with reduced bone mass.

Bisphosphonates

Bisphosphonates are stable analogues of pyrophosphate which bind to the bone surface and inhibit osteoclastic activity. Disodium etidronate has been shown to increase bone mineral density in women with spinal osteoporosis compared with placebo-treated controls, who lost bone density[219,220]. The incidence of new fractures in etidronate-treated women in one study[219] was less than that in controls. Etidronate may be of use in the treatment of steroid-induced osteoporosis (Figure 6.9)[221].

Newer and more potent bisphosphonates, such as 3-amino-1-hydroxypropylidene-1,1-bisphosphonate (APD or pamidronate) and alendronate have been developed[220]. In an early study[222], pamidronate given continuously was shown to cause a mean rise in lumbar bone density of approximately 3% per year although, in some patients, the bone mineral density increased by 50% after 4 years of treatment. A double-blind placebo-controlled study[223] of 48 postmenopausal women over 2 years indicated that pamidronate 150 mg/day increased the bone mineral density of the lumbar spine, femoral trochanter and total body.

There have been concerns that continuous use of pamidronate will halt bone remodeling, which will lead to poor microfracture repair and an increase in fracture rate. Intermittent regimens of treatment have been proposed as a method of allowing uncoupling of bone resorption and formation, and intermittent phases of positive bone balance. In a recent 2-year, prospective, double-blind study[224], 125 women were randomized to receive either oral pamidronate 300 mg/day for 4 out of every 12 weeks, oral pamidronate 150 mg/day for 4 out of every 8 weeks, or placebo. Bone mineral density at the lumbar spine and femoral neck increased significantly in the drug-treated women, but fell in women receiving placebo. There were no differences in effect on bone mineral density between the two dose regimens, but withdrawal from the study due to side-effects was nearly three times more common in women receiving the 300 mg/day regimen. In women taking oral pamidronate 150 mg/day for 4 out of every 8 weeks, the drop-out rate because of side-effects was comparable to that with placebo.

Alendronate has been reported to preserve bone mineral density, reduce vertebral and hip fracture risk, and be well tolerated in women with low bone mineral density in recent large prospective studies[225-227]. In the multicenter, randomized, double-blind, placebo-controlled, 2-year study of Chesnut and co-workers[226], 188 postmenopausal women, aged 42–75 years and with low bone mineral density of the lumbar spine, were randomized to receive placebo or one of five alendronate treatment regimens. Alendronate produced significant reductions in markers of bone resorption and formation, and significantly increased bone mineral density at the lumbar spine, hip and total body compared with decreases (significant at lumbar spine) in those receiving placebo. The mean changes in bone mineral density over 24 months with alendronate 10 mg were +7.21% for the lumbar spine, +5.27% for total hip and +2.53% for total body (all $p < 0.01$) compared with changes of –1.35%, –1.20% and –0.31%, respectively, with placebo.

More recently, the results of a randomized placebo-controlled study of the effects of alendronate on fracture risk in women aged 55–81 years, who had at least one vertebral fracture at recruitment, were reported (Fracture Intervention Trial Research Group[227]). A total of 2027 women were randomized to receive either placebo or alendronate (5 mg/day for 2 years followed by 10 mg/day for 1 year). Follow-up radiographs were obtained from 98% of surviving participants (1964 women). The relative risk of one or more new morphometric vertebral fractures for women receiving alendronate was 0.53 (95% CI 0.27–0.72), and the relative risk of hip and wrist fracture were 0.49 (95% CI 0.23–0.99) and 0.52 (95% CI 0.31–0.87), respectively.

Anabolic steroids

It is not known how anabolic steroids produce their effects on bone. It has been postulated that they have a direct effect on osteoblasts or their precursors and/or act to prevent bone resorption. There is evidence in vitro for the former effect[228]. It has recently been suggested that the increase in muscle mass induced by anabolic steroids is partly responsible for increases in bone mineral density[229].

Nandrolone has been shown to increase bone mineral content by 6% in 11 patients treated for 2 years[230]. In another study[231], 21 patients treated with stanozolol showed a mean increase of 4.4% over 29 months compared with 17 placebo patients whose bone mineral density did not change.

Chesnut and colleagues[232] studied 13 postmenopausal women taking methandrostenolone and compared the changes in total body calcium, using neutron activation, with 13 women taking placebo for 2½ years. The total body calcium fell by 3% in the placebo group and rose by 2% in the drug-treated women. The rise occurred during the first year of treatment, after which a plateau was reached. A similar study by Aloia and co-workers[233] found an initial rise in total body calcium over 6 months that was not sustained over 2 years.

Erdtsieck and colleagues[229] studied bone mineral density changes in the distal radius in women taking HRT with and without additional nandrolone decanoate for 3 years, and followed them for a further year after cessation of treatment. Bone mineral density increased more in the double-therapy group, but fell by equal rates in both groups after stopping treatment. Therefore, the increase in bone mineral density seen at the start of treatment with anabolic steroids may not be maintained with long-term treatment and may be reversed on treatment withdrawal.

Anabolic steroids in the currently used dosage regimens are inappropriate for long-term use as they produce an unfavorable lipid profile if given orally. Parenteral administration may avoid this metabolic complication, but induces increased insulin resistance[234], which is a major cardiovascular risk factor[235]. In the elderly, fluid retention due to anabolic steroid administration may increase the risk of cardiac failure.

Fluoride

Fluoride appears to stimulate new bone formation, probably by stimulation of proliferation and differentiation of committed osteoblast precursors, or by a direct action on osteoblasts. Several reports show that sodium fluoride is capable of increasing trabecular bone density[236–239], particularly in the spine. However, in one study[237], this was not associated with a reduction in vertebral fracture incidence. There are also reports that fluoride treatment results in an increased incidence of hip fracture[240]. The calcium balance appears to be unchanged in women taking fluoride, and it is possible that bone is redistributed from the hip and other sites to the spine. An alternative explanation may be that the structural quality of fluoridated hydroxyapatite is poor (Figure 6.10).

The response to fluoride varies considerably from one patient to another. Those with younger bone show the least response[238], perhaps because bone cell activity in these subjects is already high and, therefore, less able to be increased. Upper gastrointestinal side-effects may develop in patients taking fluoride, particularly those using non-enteric coated preparations. These effects usually abate after a short break in treatment. Approximately 25% of patients develop pseudoarthritic pains in the joints of the lower limb. The mechanism of this side-effect is not known, but it is often associated with high serum fluoride levels and a raised alkaline phosphate level. The pains usually disappear after a few weeks off therapy, and may be avoided when treatment is recommenced by lowering the dose and carefully monitoring the serum fluoride and alkaline phosphate.

Given the narrow therapeutic window, side-effects and concerns over femoral neck fracture, it is recommended that treatment of osteoporosis with fluoride be undertaken only in specialist centers.

Combined treatment and ADFR

'Activate, depress, free and repeat' (ADFR) regimens have recently been developed and, theoretically, may provide a means to increase bone mineral density more than with single-treatment methods[241]. A drug capable of stimulating bone formation is given first, followed by an agent that depresses bone resorption. It is postulated that, during the 'free' period, the former steadily increases bone at each remodeling site. The cycle is repeated as required.

Most studies involving this method have used phosphate as the activating agent in combination with calcitonin or etidronate[242,243]. It appears that phosphate/etidronate combinations achieve no better results than cyclical etidronate alone, perhaps because the long skeletal half-life of the bisphosphonates renders them unsuitable candidates for ADFR regimens. A recent 3-year study[244] of an ADFR regimen using triiodothyronine as activator and etidronate as suppressor showed no preservation of bone density in 18 women treated for 3 years. Another study using parathyroid hormone as the activator and calcitonin as the suppressor has shown preliminary results that are encouraging[245].

Lindsay and colleagues[246] conducted a 3-year randomized controlled trial to examine the effects of 1–34 human parathyroid hormone (hPTH (1–34), 400 U/25 mg daily subcutaneously) in 17 postmenopausal women with osteoporosis taking HRT. A control group of 17 women took HRT alone. The women taking HRT and hPTH (1–34) showed continuous increases in vertebral bone mineral density over the 3 years whereas no significant changes were seen in the controls. The total increase in vertebral bone mineral density was 13.0% ($p < 0.001$), 2.7% at the hip ($p = 0.05$) and 8.0% for total body bone mineral ($p = 0.002$). No loss of bone mass was found at any skeletal site. Increased bone mass was associated with a reduction in the rate of vertebral fractures.

Vitamin D

There is little evidence that vitamin D or its analogues are of any value in the treatment or prevention of osteoporosis for the majority of women in Western societies[247-249], although large studies in Japan have shown fracture incidence reduction; in addition, vitamin D supplementation may be beneficial for elderly or institutionalized vitamin D-deficient women[250]. A study[251] of a Western population using 200 IU of vitamin D for 2 years showed preservation of bone mineral density in the spine, but not in the femoral neck. It is likely that the dosages of vitamin D metabolites necessary to produce a positive effect on bone are associated with toxicity. New vitamin D metabolites may avoid such side-effects and studies are awaited with interest.

Calcium

It appears that, for the majority of adults following a healthy diet, calcium supplementation has little or no effect on bone mineral density. There have been few satisfactory prospective studies of the effects of calcium supplementation on bone density independent of increased energy intake. Although, in one study[252], a particular calcium salt had some effect on bone mineral density when given to older women with very low calcium intake, there is no good evidence that increasing dietary calcium intake to >500 mg/day in adults has any significant benefit (Figures 6.10 and 6.11). A recent trial[253] reported a reduction of lumbar spine bone loss after 1 year, but no subsequent reduction during a further 3 years of treatment. It is likely that any small increase in bone density achieved by alterations in dietary calcium intake is insufficient to prevent the rapid decrease that occurs in women around the time of the menopause. In summary, the evidence for increasing calcium intake to benefit the skeleton remains controversial[94,254]. However, given in conjunction with vitamin D, it probably has a useful role in the management of osteoporosis in the elderly[250].

Exercise

In a previously sedentary patient, a program of regular exercise is not only likely to increase bone mineral density, but will probably also improve dexterity and muscle mass, thereby reducing the chances of serious fracture should a fall occur. Regular weight-bearing exercise produces a small benefit to bone density in postmenopausal women[84,255-257] but, by itself, is unable to prevent normal postmenopausal bone loss. A recent report[257] suggested that there may be a protective effect of lifelong and current exercise on hip bone mineral density in postmenopausal women, but no effect on fracture risk. Furthermore, it has been shown that the benefits gained by exercise are rapidly lost if a sedentary lifestyle is resumed[258]. Thus, exercise should be regarded as an adjuvant, rather than alternative, to active treatment for osteoporosis.

Patients who are not osteoporotic should be encouraged to take up exercise that puts stress on weight-bearing bones, such as the spine or hip, as is appropriate to their cardiovascular fitness. Good examples are walking, jogging and playing tennis. In established osteoporotics, exercise that involves jarring movements and flexion of the back should be avoided; the emphasis should be towards activity that encourages flexibility.

Prevention of falls

Falls in the elderly are common, and occur more frequently in women and with advancing age[259]. Although it has been estimated that, in the general postmenopausal population, only 2–5% of falls result in fracture[260], and many of the predisposing factors are unavoidable (such as chronic ill health and cognitive impairment), strategies aimed at reducing avoidable risks may be expected to reduce the incidence of fracture. Such risks include the use of sedatives (including alcohol), wearing inappropriate footwear, hazardous home arrangements and travelling in poor weather conditions.

Hip protectors

An additional approach for reducing hip fracture is to prevent direct trauma to the hip with the use of hip protectors with rigid inserts (Figure 6.11). As the incidence of fracture following falls on the hip has been estimated to be much higher, approximately 24%, among nursing-home residents than in the general population, this group of subjects may benefit most from this form of treatment. In a study of nursing-home residents, Lauritzen and co-workers[261] showed that the relative risk of hip fracture among women and men using hip protectors was 0.44 (95% CI 0.21–0.94).

7 Conclusions

Diagnosis and screening

Osteoporosis manifests itself clinically as fractures but, by the time the bone density has fallen to levels that predispose to fracture with minimal trauma, the treatment options are limited. Modern management aims to identify those patients who are at risk of developing fracture in the future.

Several studies have shown that the presence of risk factors in a given individual is not a good predictor of bone density[85,262–267]. Therefore, at present, the risk of fracture must be predicted by measuring bone mineral density or identifying other factors that predispose to falls. There have been no satisfactory studies of the effects of screening the whole population for osteoporosis. Thus, it is not possible to conclude whether screening is of value in predicting osteoporotic fracture in the absence of data.

It is also false to assume that screening is of no value on the basis of some studies which have shown that long-term compliance with the most commonly used treatment for osteoporosis, namely, HRT, is poor[268,269]. The majority of postmenopausal women presently seek HRT for the relief of climacteric symptoms[270] and not for the treatment of osteoporosis. It is not known what the long-term compliance will be in a population receiving HRT primarily for its effects on bone. In the absence of evidence for or against screening, our current policy for patients presenting at menopause clinics is to measure the bone mineral density at the hip or spine, using DEXA or CT, of those patients who present with osteoporotic fracture or risk factors for fracture, or of those women who request HRT solely for the treatment or prevention of osteoporosis.

Treatment

Estrogen replacement therapy is the method of treatment and prevention of osteoporosis that has been the most studied, and is considered by many to be the drug of first choice for postmenopausal women. Bisphosphonates and calcitonin are suitable alternative drugs to prevent bone resorption in those women who are reluctant to take HRT, but it should be made clear to these patients that such treatments have none of the beneficial effects of HRT in reducing the mortality of myocardial infarction[271] or the incidence of stroke[272]. Patients with severe osteoporosis may benefit from a combination of one drug to prevent resorption and another to stimulate bone formation. Of the latter category, only anabolic steroids have been studied sufficiently to recommend their general use. However, they should only be prescribed with the supervision of a physician who has experience of this method of treatment. As it is likely that a small number of women will lose bone density while taking so-called standard bone-preserving doses of HRT, it is advisable to repeat bone mineral density measurements in women who are known to have very low bone density before treatment. Unfortunately, the optimal management of the patient whose bone density falls while receiving standard-dose HRT is unknown. Two possible strategies are to increase the dose of estrogen or to use combination treatment.

The duration of therapy for the prevention or treatment of osteoporosis must be tailored to the needs of the given patient. Decisions concerning the duration of treatment may be guided by bone mineral density measurements. Thus, the patient who has been receiving HRT for 10 years and who is contemplating stopping therapy may be advised not to do so if her bone mineral density estimation is significantly below that of her age-matched peers.

If bone density measurements are unavailable and general strategies of therapy must be adopted, then 5–10 years is generally considered to be the minimal duration of treatment necessary to significantly reduce the risk of fracture in at-risk populations. However, such general guidelines are a poor substitute for therapy which is determined by the requirements of the given individual. It is hoped that methods of measuring bone density, and predicting the response of bone to aging and the menopause will become more widely available in the future.

References

1. Melton LJ IIIrd. Etiology, diagnosis and management. In: Riggs B, Melton LI, eds. *Epidemiology of Fractures*. New York: Raven Press, 1988:133–54

2. Consensus conference: Osteoporosis. *J Am Med Assoc* 1984;252:99–802

3. Melton LJ IIIrd. Hip fractures: A worldwide problem today and tomorrow. *Bone* 1993;14(Suppl 1): S1–8

4. Grimley Evans J. The significance of osteoporosis. In: Smith R, ed. *Osteoporosis*. London: Royal College of Physicians, 1990:1–8

5. Alffram PS, Bauer G. Epidemiology of fractures of the forearm. *J Bone Joint Surg* 1962;44(A):105–14

6. Office of Population Censuses and Surveys. *Hospital Inpatient Enquiry, 1985*. London: HMSO, 1987

7. Spector TD, Cooper C, Fenton Lewis A. Trends in admissions for hip fracture in England and Wales. *BMJ* 1990;300:173–4

8. Boyce WJ, Vessey MP. Rising incidence of fracture of the proximal femur. *Lancet* 1985;i:150–1

9. Lindsay R, Hart DM. The minimum effective dose of estrogen for prevention of postmenopausal bone loss. *Obstet Gynecol* 1984;63:759–63

10. Grimley Evans J, Prudham D, Wandles I. A prospective study of fractured proximal femur: Incidence and outcome. *Public Health* (London) 1979;93:235–41

11. Nordin BEC, Crilly RG, Smith DA. Osteoporosis. In: Nordin B, ed. *Metabolic Bone and Stone Disease*. Edinburgh: Churchill Livingstone, 1984:1–70

12. Law MR, Wald NJ, Meade TW. Strategies for prevention of osteoporosis and hip fracture. *BMJ* 1991;303:453–9

13. Miller CW. Survival and ambulation following hip fractures. *J Bone Joint Surg* 1978;60(A):930–4

14. Riggs BL, Melton LJ. Involutional osteoporosis. *N Engl J Med* 1986;314:1676–86

15. Chrischilles E, Shireman T, Wallace R. Costs and health effects of osteoporotic fractures. *Bone* 1994; 15:377–86

16. Smith RW, Risek J. Epidemiological studies of osteoporosis in women of Puerto Rico and southwestern Michigan. *Clin Orthop* 1962;45:31–48

17. Lindsay R. Pathogenesis, detection and prevention of postmenopausal osteoporosis. In: Studd J, Whitehead M, eds. *The Menopause*. Oxford: Blackwell Scientific Publications, 1988:156–67

18. Obrant K, Bengnér U, Johnell O, *et al.* Increasing age-adjusted risk of fragility fractures: A sign of increasing osteoporosis in successive generations? *Calcif Tissue Int* 1989;44:157–67

19. Leichter I, Margulies JY, Weinreb A, *et al.* The relationship between bone density, mineral content, and mechanical strength in the femoral neck. *Clin Orthop* 1982;163:272–81

20. Dalen N, Hellstrom L-G, Jacobson B. Bone mineral content and mechanical strength of the femoral neck. *Acta Orthop Scand* 1976;47:503–8

21. Hui SL, Slemenda CW, Johnson CC Jr. Age and bone mass as predictors of fracture in a prospective study. *J Clin Invest* 1988;81:1804–9

22. Gardsell P, Johnell O, Nilsson BE. Predicting fractures in women using forearm bone densitometry. *Calcif Tissue Int* 1989;44:355–61

23. Browner WS, Cummings SR, Genat HK. Bone mineral density and fractures of the wrist and humerus in elderly women: A prospective study. *J Bone Miner Res* 1989;4(Suppl):S171

24. Cummings SR, Black DM, Nevitt MC, *et al.* Appendicular bone density and age predict hip fractures in women. *J Am Med Assoc* 1990;263:665–8

25. Ott SM, Kilcoyne RF, Chesnut CH IIIrd. Ability of four different techniques of measuring bone mass to diagnose vertebral fractures in postmenopausal women. *J Bone Miner Res* 1987;2:201–10

26. Stevenson JC, Allen PR, Abeyesekera G, Hill PA. Osteoporosis with hip fracture: Changes in calcium regulating hormones. *Eur J Clin Invest* 1986;16:357–60

27. Mazess RB, Barden H, Ettinger M, Schultz E. Bone density of the radius, spine, and proximal femur in osteopororsis. *J Bone Miner Res* 1988;3:13–8

28. Riggs BL, Wahner HW, Seeman E, *et al.* Changes in bone mineral density of the proximal femur and spine with aging. Differences between the postmenopausal and senile osteoporosis syndromes. *J Clin Invest* 1982;70:716–23

29 Nordin BEC, Wishart JM, Horowitz M, *et al.* The relation between forearm and vertebral mineral density and fractures in postmenopausal women. *Bone Miner* 1988;5:21–33

30. Eastell R, Wahner HW, O'Fallon WM, *et al.* Unequal decrease in bone density of lumbar spine and ultradistal radius in Colles' and vertebral fracture syndromes. *J Clin Invest* 1989;83:168–74

31. Marshall D, Johnell O, Wedel H. Meta-analysis of how well measures of bone mineral density predict occurrence of osteoporotic fractures. *BMJ* 1996;312:1254–9

32. Boonen S, Koutri R, Dequeker J, *et al.* Measurement of femoral geometry in type I and type II osteoporosis: Differences in hip axis length consistent with heterogeneity in the pathogenesis of osteoporotic fractures. *J Bone Miner Res* 1995;10:1908–12

33. Chevalley T, Rizzoli R, Nydegger V, *et al.* Preferential low bone mineral density of the femoral neck in patients with a recent fracture of the proximal femur. *Osteoporos Int* 1991;1:147–54

34. Eriksson SAV, Wilde TL. Bone mass in women with hip fracture. *Orthop Scand* 1988;59:19–23

35. Bohr H, Schaadt O. Bone mineral content of femoral bone and the lumbar spine measured in women with fracture of the femoral neck by dual photon absorptiometry. *Clin Orthop* 1983;179:240–5

36. Davis JW, Vogel JM, Ross PD, Wasnich RD. Disease versus etiology: The distinction should not be lost in the analysis. *J Nucl Med* 1989;112:1273–6

37. Rose G. Sick individuals and sick populations. *Int J Epidemiol* 1985;14:32–8

38. Stevenson JC, Marsh MS. Preventing osteoporosis [Letter]. *BMJ* 1991;303:920–1

39. Ross PD, Wasnich RD, McClean CJ, *et al.* A model for estimating the potential costs and savings of osteoporosis prevention strategies. *Bone* 1988;9:337–47

40. Cummings SR. Are patients with hip fractures more osteoporotic? *Am J Med* 1985;78:487–94

41. Winner SJ, Morgan A, Grimley Evans J. Perimenopausal risk of falling and incidence of distal forearm fracture. *BMJ* 1989;298:1486–8

42. Dargent-Molina P, Favier F, Grandjean H, *et al.* Fall-related factors and risk of hip fracture: The EPIDOS prospective study. Epidémiologie de l'ostéoporose. *Lancet* 1996;348:145–9

43. Kanis JA, Aaron J, Thavarajah M, *et al.* Osteoporosis: Causes and therapeutic implications. In: Smith R, ed. *Osteoporosis*. London: Royal College of Physicians, 1990:45–56

44. Nevitt MC, Cummings SR, for The Study of Osteoporotic Fractures Research Group. Type of fall and risk of hip and wrist fractures: The study of osteoporotic fractures. *J Am Geriatr Soc* 1993;41:1226–34

45. Owen M, Ashton B. Osteogenic differentiation of different skeletal cell populations. In: Ali S, ed. *Cell Mediated Calcification and Matrix Vesicles*. Amsterdam: Elsevier, 1986:279–84

46. Anderson HC. Matrix vesicle calcification: Review and update. *Bone and Mineral Research.* Amsterdam: Elsevier, 1985:109–49

47. Schneider GB, Relfson M, Nicolas J. Pluripotential hemopoietic stem cells give rise to osteoclasts. *Am J Anat* 1986;177:505–12

48. Marchisio PC, Cirillo D, Naldini L, *et al.* Cell substratum interaction of cultured avian osteoclasts is mediated by specific adhesion structures. *J Cell Biol* 1984;99:1696–705

49. Vaes G. Cellular biology and biochemical mechanisms of bone resorption. *Clin Orthop* 1988;231: 239–71

50. Russell RGG, Caswell AM, Hearn PR, Sharrard RM. Calcium in mineralised tissues and pathological calcification. *Br Med Bull* 1986;42:435–46

51. Yamaguchi K, Croucher PI, Compston JE. Comparison between the lengths of individual osteoid seams and resorption cavities in human iliac crest cancellous bone. *Bone & Miner* 1993;23:27–33

52. Jones SJ, Boyd A. Experimental study of changes in osteoblastic shape induced by calcitonin and parathyroid extract in an organ culture system. *Cell Tissue Res* 1976;169:449–55

53. Russell RGG. Bone cell biology: The role of cytokines and other mediators. In: Smith R, ed. *Osteoporosis*. London: Royal College of Physicians, 1990:9–33

54. Komm BS, Sheetz BS, Baker M, *et al.* Bone-related cells in culture express putative oestrogen receptor mRNA and ^{125}I–17β-oestradiol binding. *J Bone Miner Res* 1987;2(Suppl 1):237

55. Eriksen EF, Berg BJ, Graham ML, *et al.* Evidence of oestrogen receptors in human bone cells. *J Bone Miner Res* 1987;2(Suppl 1):238

56. Coffer AI, Lewis KM, Brokas AJ, King RJB. Monoclonal antibodies against a component related to soluble estrogen receptor. *Cancer Res* 1985; 45:3686–93

57. Colston KW, King RWB, Hayward J, *et al.* Estrogen receptors and human bone cells: Immunocytochemical studies. *J Bone Miner Res* 1989;4,625–31

58. Russell RGG, Bunning RAD, Hughes DE, Gowen M. Humoral and local factors affecting bone formation and resorption. In: Stevenson J, ed. *New Techniques in Metabolic Bone Disease.* London: Wright, 1990:1–20

59. Stevenson JC, Abeyasekera G, Hillyard CJ, *et al.* Regulation of calcium-regulating hormones by exogenous sex steroids in early postmenopause. *Eur J Clin Invest* 1983;13:481–7

60. Stevenson JC, Abeyasekera G, Hillyard CJ, *et al.* Calcitonin and the calcium-regulating hormones in

postmenopausal women: Effect of oestrogens. *Lancet* 1981;i:693–5

61. Delorme ML, Digioia Y, Fandard J, *et al.* Oestrogens et calcitonie. *Ann d'Endo* 1976;37:503–4

62. Hillyard CJ, Stevenson JC, MacIntyre I. Relative deficiency of plasma–calcitonin in normal women. *Lancet* 1978;i:961–2

63. Tiegs RD, Barta J, Heath H. Does oral contraceptive therapy affect calcitonin secretion in premenopausal women? *Presented at The Endocrine Society 67th Annual General Meeting,* 1985:50

64. Taggart HM, Chesnut CH IIIrd, Ivey JL, *et al.* Deficient calcitonin response to calcium stimulation in postmenopausal osteoporosis. *Lancet* 1982; i:475–8

65. Tiegs RD, Body JJ, Wahner HW, *et al.* Calcitonin secretion in postmenopausal osteoporosis. *N Engl J Med* 1985;312:1097–100

66. Pacifici R, Rifas L, Teitelbaum S, *et al.* Spontaneous release of interleukin-1 from human blood monocytes reflects bone formation in idiopathic bone osteoporosis. *Proceedings of the National Academy of Sciences of the US* 1987;84:4616–20

67. Ralston SH. Analysis of gene expression in human bone biopsies by polymerase chain reaction: Evidence for enhanced cytokine expression in postmenopausal osteoporosis. *J Bone Miner Res* 1994;8:83–90

68. Bertolini DR, Nedwin GE, Bringman TS, *et al.* Stimulation of bone resorption and inhibition of bone formation *in vitro* by human tumor necrosis factors. *Nature* 1986;319:516–21

69. Kimble RB, Matayoshi AB, Vannice JL, *et al.* Simultaneous block of interleukin-1 and tumor necrosis factor is required to completely prevent bone loss in the early postovariectomy period. *Endocrinology* 1995;136:3054–61

70. Peterlik M, Hoffmann O, Swetly P, *et al.* Recombinant gamma-interferon inhibits prostaglandin-mediated and parathyroid hormone-induced bone resorption in cultured neonatal mouse calvaria. *FEBS Lett* 1985;185:287–90

71. Ross R. Platelet-derived growth factor. *Lancet* 1989;i:1312–15

72. Kalu DN, Salerno E, Higami Y, *et al.* In vivo effects of transforming growth factor-beta 2 in ovariectomized rats. *Bone & Miner* 1993;22:209-20

73. Hughes DE, Dai A, Tiffee JC, *et al.* Estrogen promotes apoptosis of murine osteoclasts mediated by TGF-beta. *Nature Med* 1996;2:1132–6

74. Raisz LG, Martin TJ. Prostaglandins in bone and mineral metabolism. In: Peck W, ed. *Bone and Mineral Research.* Amsterdam: Elsevier, 1984

75. Ibbotson KJ, Twardzic DR, D'Souza SM, *et al.* Stimulation of bone resorption *in vitro* by synthetic transforming growth factor-alpha. *Science* 1985; 228:1007

76. Feyen JHM, Raisz LG. Prostaglandin production by calvariae from sham-operated and oophorectomised rats: Effect of 17β-estradiol *in vivo. Endocrinology* 1987;121:819–21

77. Ralston SH, Ho LP, Helfrich MH, *et al.* Nitric oxide: A cytokine-induced regulator of bone resorption. *J Bone Miner Res* 1995;10:1040–9

78. Ralston SH, Todd D, Helfrich MH, *et al.* Human osteoblast-like cells produce nitric oxide and express inducible nitric oxide synthase. *Endocrinology* 1994;135:330–6

79. Ralston SH, Grabowski PS. Mechanisms of cytokine-induced bone resorption; role of nitric oxide, cyclic guanosine monophosphate and prostaglandins. *Bone* 1996;19:29–33

80. Evans DM, Ralston SH. Nitric oxide and bone. *J Bone Miner Res* 1996;11:300–5

81. Schlesinger PH, Mattsson JP, Blair HC. Osteoclastic acid transport: Mechanism and implications for physiological and pharmacological regulation. *Miner Electrolyte Metab* 1994;20:31–9

82. David P, Nguyen H, Barbier A, Baron R. The bisphosphonate tiludronate is a potent inhibitor of the osteoclast vacuolar H(+)-ATPase. *J Bone Miner Res* 1996;11:1498–507

83. Pacifici R. Estrogen, cytokines, and pathogenesis of postmenopausal osteoporosis. *J Bone Miner Res* 1996;11:1043–51

84. Wasnich RD, Ross PD, Davis JW, Vogel JM. A comparison of single and multisite BMC measurements for assessment of spine fracture probability. *J Nucl Med* 1989;30:1166–71

85. Stevenson JC, Lees B, Devenport M, et al. Determinants of bone density in normal women: Risk factors for future osteoporosis? *BMJ* 1989;298:924–8

86. Thomsen K, Gotfredsen A, Christiansen C. Is postmenopausal bone loss an age-related phenomenon? *Calcif Tissue Int* 1986;39:132–27

87. Guesens P, Dequeker J, Verstraeten A, Nijs J. Age, sex- and menopause-related changes of vertebral and peripheral bone: Population study using dual-photon absorptiometry and radiogrammetry. *J Nucl Med* 1986;27:1540–9

88. Smith DM, Nance WE, Kang KW, et al. Genetic factors in determining bone mass. *J Clin Invest* 1973;52:2800–08

89. Seeman E, Tsalamandris C, Formica C, et al. Reduced femoral neck bone density in the daughters of women with hip fractures: The role of low peak bone density in the pathogenesis of osteoporosis. *J Bone Miner Res* 1994;9:739–43

90. Cohn SH, Abesamis C, Yamasura S, et al. Comparative skeletal mass and radial bone mineral content in black and white women. *Metabolism* 1977;26: 171–8

91. Kanders B, Lindsay R, Dempster DW, et al. Determinants of bone mass in young healthy women. In: Christiansen C, ed. *Osteoporosis.* Aalborg: Stiftsbogtrykkeri, 1984:337–40

92. Sandler RB, Slemenda CW, LaPorte RE, et al. Postmenopausal bone density and milk consumption in childhood and adolescence. *Am J Clin Nutr* 1985;42:270–4

93. Soroko S, Holbrook TL, Edelstein S, Barrett-Connor E. Lifetime milk consumption and bone mineral density in older women. *Am J Pub Health* 1994;84:1319–22

94. Kanis JA, Passmore R. Calcium supplementation of the diet-1. *BMJ* 1989;298:137–40

95. Greendale GA, Barrett-Connor E, Edelstein S, et al. Lifetime leisure exercise and osteoporosis. The Rancho Bernardo study. *Am J Epidemiol* 1995;141:951–9

96. Jaglal SB, Kreiger N, Darlington GA. Lifetime occupational physical activity and risk of hip fracture in women. *Ann Epidemiol* 1995;5:321–4

97. Cooper C, Cawley M, Bhalla A, et al. Childhood growth, physical activity, and peak bone mass in women. *J Bone Miner Res* 1995;10:940–7

98. Lloyd T, Myers C, Buchanan JR, Demers LM. Collegiate women athletes with irregular menses during adolescence have decreased bone density. *Obstet Gynecol* 1988;72:639–42

99. Lindberg JS, Fears WB, Hunt MM, et al. Exercise induced amenorrhea and bone density. *Ann Intern Med* 1984;101:258–60

100. Drinkwater BL, Nilson K, Chesnut CH IIIrd, et al. Bone mineral density of amenorrheic and eumenorrheic athletes. *N Engl J Med* 1984;311:277–81

101. Slemender CW, Hui SL, Longcope C, Johnson CC. Cigarette smoking. Obesity and bone mass. *J Bone Miner Res* 1989;4:737–41

102. Baron BA. Smoking and estrogen-related disease. *Am J Epidemiol* 1984;119:9–22

103. Rigotti NA. Cigarette smoking and body weight. *N Engl J Med* 1989;320:931–3

104. Hopper JL, Seeman E. The bone density of female twins discordant for tobacco use. *N Engl J Med* 1994;330:387–92

105. Saville PD. Changes in bone mass with age and alcoholism. *J Bone Joint Surg* 1965;47:492–9

106. De Vernejoul MC, Bielakoff J, Herve M, *et al.* Evidence for defective osteoblastic function. A role for alcohol and tobacco consumption in osteoporosis in middle aged men. *Clin Orthop* 1983;179: 107–15

107. Tuppurainen M, Kroger H, Honkanen R, *et al.* Risks of perimenopausal fractures – a prospective population-based study. *Acta Obstet Gynecol Scand* 1995;74:624–8

108. Murphy S, Shaw KT, May H, Compston JE. Parity and bone density in middle age women. *Osteoporos Int* 1994;4:162–6

109. Riggs BL, Wahner HW, Dunn WL, *et al.* Differential changes in bone mineral density of the appendicular and axial skeleton with aging: Relationship to spinal osteoporosis. *J Clin Invest* 1981;67:328–35

110. Nordin BEC, Marshall DH, Francis RM, Crilly RG. The effect of sex steroid and corticosteroid hormones on bone. *J Steroid Biochem* 1981;15:171–4

111. Abdallah H, Hart DM, Lindsay R. Differential bone loss and effects of long-term oestrogen therapy according to time of introduction of therapy after oophorectomy. In: Christiansen C, Arnaud C, Nordin B, *et al.*, eds. *Osteoporosis.* Glostrup: Glostrup Hospital, 1984:621–3

112. Krolner B, Nielsen SP. Bone mineral content of the lumbar spine in normal and osteoporotic women: Cross-sectional and longitudinal studies. *Clin Sci* 1982;62:329–36

113. Riggs BL, Jowsey J, Kelly PJ, *et al.* Effect of sex hormones on bone in primary osteoporosis. *J Clin Invest* 1969;48:1065–72

114. Nordin BEC, Aaron J, Speed R, Crilly RG. Bone formation and resorption as the determinants of trabecular bone volume in postmenopausal osteoporosis. *Lancet* 1981;ii:277–9

115. Heaney RP, Recker RR, Saville PD. Menopausal changes in bone remodelling. *J Lab Clin Med* 1978; 92:964–70

116. Hansen JW, Gordan GS, Prussin SG. Direct measurement of osteolysis in man. *J Clin Invest* 1973; 52:304–15

117. Ettinger B, Genant HK, Cann CE. Postmenopausal bone loss is prevented by treatment with low dosage estrogen with calcium. *Ann Intern Med* 1987; 106:40–5

118. Stevenson JC, Lees B, Banks LM, Whitehead MI. Assessment of therapeutic options for prevention of bone loss. In: Christiansen C, Johansen J, Riis BJ, eds. *Osteoporosis.* Viborg: Norhaven Bogtrykken A/S, 1987:392–3

119. Genant HK, Cann CE, Ettinger B, Gordan GS. Quantitative computed tomography of vertebral spongiosa: A sensitive method of detecting early bone loss after oophorectomy. *Ann Intern Med* 1982;97:699–705

120. Christiansen C, Christiansen MS, Transbøl I. Bone mass in postmenopausal women after withdrawal of oestrogen replacement therapy. *Lancet* 1981;i: 459–61

121. Stevenson JC, Banks LM, Spinks TJ, *et al.* Regional and total skeletal measurements in the early postmenopause. *J Clin Invest* 1987;80:258–62

122. Lindsay R, Hart DM, Aitken JM, *et al.* Long-term prevention of postmenopausal osteoporosis by oestrogen. *Lancet* 1976;i:1038–41

123. Riis BJ. The role of bone loss. *Am J Med* 1995;98: 29S–32S

124. Christiansen C. What should be done at the time of menopause? *Am J Med* 1995;98:56S–9S

125. Christiansen C, Riis BJ, Rødbro P. Prediction of rapid bone loss in postmenopausal women. *Lancet* 1987;i:1105–7

126. Poortman J, Thijssen JHH, de Waard F. Plasma oestrone, oestradiol and androstanedione levels in postmenopausal women: Relation to body weight and height. *Maturitas* 1981;3:65–71

127. MacDonald PC, Edman CD, Hemsell DL, *et al*. Effect of obesity on conversion of plasma androstanedione to estrone in postmenopausal women with and without endometrial cancer. *Am J Obstet Gynecol* 1978;130:448–55

128. Christiansen C. Prophylactic treatment for age-related bone loss in women. *Proceedings of the International Symposium on Osteoporosis, Copenhagen,* 1984;2:587–93

129. Johnston CC Jr, Hui SL, Witt RM, *et al*. Early menopausal changes in bone mass and sex steroids. *J Clin Endocrinol Metab* 1985;61:905–11

130. Slemender C, Hui SL, Longcope C, Johnston CC. Sex steroids and bone mass: A study about the time of menopause. *J Clin Invest* 1987;80:1261–9

131. Clements D, Compston JE, Evans C, Evans WD. Bone loss in normal British women; a 5-year follow-up. *Br J Radiol* 1993;66:1134–7

132. Pugh JW, Rose RM, Radin EL. Elastic and viscoelastic properties of bone. *J Biomech* 1973;6:475–85

133. Compston JE, Mellish RWE, Garrahan NJ. Age-related changes in the iliac crest trabecular microanatomic bone structure in man. *Bone* 1978; 8:289–92

134. Compston JE. Structural mechanisms of trabecular bone loss. In: Smith R, ed. *Osteoporosis*. London: Royal College of Physicians, 1990:35–43

135. Croucher PI, Garrahan NJ, Compston JE. Assessment of cancellous bone structure: Comparison of strut analysis, trabecular bone pattern factor, and marrow space star volume. *J Bone Miner Res* 1996;11:955–61

136. Peacock M. Hypercalcaemia and calcium homeostasis. *Metab Bone Dis Rel Res* 1980;2:143–50

137. Marshall RW, Francis RM, Hodgkinson A. Plasma total and ionised calcium, albumin and globulin concentrations in pre- and postmenopausal women and the effects of oestrogen administration. *Clin Chim Acta* 1982;122:283–7

138. Stevenson JC. Vitamin D in postmenopausal women. In: Duursma S, van der Sluys Veer J, eds. *Vitamin D*. Utrecht: Wetenschappelijke uitgerij Bunge, 1983:43–55

139. Heaney RP, Recker RR, Saville PD. Menopausal changes in calcium balance performance. *J Lab Clin Med* 1978;92:953–63

140. Riggs BL, Jowsey J, Kelley PJ, Arnaud CD. Role of hormonal factors in the pathogenesis of postmenopausal osteoporosis. *Isr J Med Sci* 1976;12: 615–9

141. Nordin BEC. Osteomalacia, osteoporosis and calcium deficiency. *Clin Orthop* 1960;17:235–57

142. Riggs BL, Melton LJ. Evidence for two distinct syndromes of involutional osteoporosis. *Am J Med* 1983;75:899–901

143. Reeve J. The use of biochemical and isotopic studies in the investigation of bone disorders. In: Stevenson J, ed. *New Techniques in Metabolic Bone Disease*. London: Wright, 1990:92–109

144. Stepan JJ, Volek V, Kolar JA. A modified inactivation inhibition method for determining the serum activity of alkaline phosphatase isoenzymes. *Clin Chim Acta* 1976;69:1–9

145. Moss DW, King EJ. Properties of alkaline phosphatase fractions separated by starch gel electrophoresis. *Biochemistry* 1962;84:192–5

146. Posen S, Neale FC, Clubb JS. Heat inactivation in the study of human alkaline phosphatases. *Ann Intern Med* 1965;62:1234–43

147. Christiansen C, Riis BJ. Risk assessment using biochemical analysis. In: Smith R, ed. *Osteoporosis*. London: Royal College of Physicians, 1990:158–61

148. Hasling C, Eriksen EF, Melkko J, *et al*. Effects of a combined estrogen–gestagen regimen on serum levels of the carboxy-terminal propeptide of human type I procollagen in osteoporosis. *J Bone Miner Res* 1991;6:1295–300

149. Brown JP, Delmas PD, Malval L, *et al*. Serum bone Gla protein: A specific marker for bone formation in postmenopausal osteoporosis. *Lancet* 1984; i:1091–3

150. Miura H, Yamamoto I, Yuu I, *et al*. Estimation of bone mineral density and bone loss by means of bone metabolic markers in postmenopausal women. *Endocrinol Jpn* 1995;42:797–802

151. Dresner-Pollak R, Parker RA, Poku M, *et al*. Biochemical markers of bone turnover reflect femoral bone loss in elderly women. *Calcif Tissue Int* 1996; 59:328–33

152. Seibel MJ, Cosman F, Shen V, *et al*. Urinary hydroxypyridinium crosslinks of collagen as markers of bone resorption and estrogen efficacy in postmenopausal osteoporosis. *J Bone Miner Res* 1993;8: 881–9

153. Schlemmer A, Hassager C, Delmas PD, Christiansen C. Urinary excretion of pyridinium cross-links in healthy women; the long-term effects of menopause and oestrogen/progesterone therapy. *Clin Endocrinol* 1994;40:777–82

154. Eastell R, Robins SP, Colwel T, *et al*. Evaluation of bone turnover in type I osteoporosis using biochemical markers specific for both bone formation and bone resorption. *Osteoporos Int* 1993;3:255–60

155. Charles P, Mosekilde L, Risteli L, *et al*. Assessment of bone remodelling using biochemical indicators of type I collagen synthesis and degradation: relation to calcium kinetics. *Bone & Miner* 1994;24:81–94

156. Valimaki MJ, Tahtela R, Jones JD, *et al*. Bone resorption in healthy and osteoporotic postmenopausal women: Comparison markers for serum carboxy-terminal telopeptide of type I collagen and urinary pyridinium cross-links. *Eur J Endocrinol* 1994;131:258–62

157. Eriksen EF, Charles P, Melsen F, *et al*. Serum markers of type I collagen formation and degradation in metabolic bone disease: Correlation with bone histomorphometry. *J Bone Miner Res* 1993;8:127–32

158. Hassager C, Jensen LT, Podenphant J, *et al*. The carboxy-terminal pyridinoline cross-linked telopeptide of type I collagen in serum as a marker of bone resorption: The effect of nandrolone decanoate and hormone replacement therapy. *Calcif Tissue Int* 1994;54:30–3

159. Khosla S, Peterson JM, Egan K, *et al*. Circulating cytokine levels in osteoporotic and normal women. *J Clin Endocrinol Metab* 1994;79:707–11

160. Bettica P, Taylor AK, Talbot J, *et al*. Clinical performances of galactosyl hydroxylysine, pyridinoline, and deoxypyridinoline in postmenopausal osteoporosis. *J Clin Endocrinol Metab* 1996;81:542–6

161. Stulberg BN, Bauer TW, Watson JT, Richmond B. Bone quality. Roentgenographic versus histologic assessment of hip bone structure. *Clin Orthop* 1989; 240:200–5

162. Hurxthal LM, Vose GP, Dotter WE. Densitometric and visual observations of spinal radiographs. *Geriatrics* 1969;24:93–106

163. Doyle FH. Involutional osteoporosis. In: MacIntyre I, ed. *Clinics in Endocrinology and Metabolism*. London: W.B. Saunders, 1972:143–67

164. Grubb SA, Jacobson PC, Aubrey BJ, *et al.* Bone density in osteoporotic women: A modified distal radius density measurement procedure to develop an 'at risk' value for use in screening women. *J Orthop Res* 1984;2:328–32

165. Borg J, Mollgaard A, Riis BJ. Single x-ray absorptiometry: Performance characteristics and comparison with single-photon absorptiometry. *Osteoporos Int* 1995;5:377–81

166. Banks LM, Stevenson JC. Developments in computerized axial tomography scanning and its use in bone disease measurement. In: Stevenson J, ed. *New Techniques in Metabolic Bone Disease.* London: Wright, 1990:138–56

167. Guglielmi G, Grimston SK, Fischer KC, Pacifici R. Osteoporosis: Diagnosis with lateral and posteroanterior dual x-ray absorptiometry compared with quantitative CT. *Radiology* 1994;192:845–50

168. Jergas M, Breitenseher M, Gluer CC, *et al.* Estimates of volumetric bone density from projectional measurements improve the discriminatory capability of dual x-ray absorptiometry. *J Bone Miner Res* 1995;10:1101–10

169. Grampp S, Jergas M, Lang P, *et al.* Quantitative CT assessment of the lumbar spine and radius in patients with osteoporosis. *Am J Roentgenol* 1996;167:133–40

170. Grampp S, Lang P, Jergas M, *et al.* Assessment of the skeletal status by peripheral quantitative computed tomography of the forearm: Short-term precision *in vivo* and comparison to dual x-ray absorptiometry. *J Bone Miner Res* 1995;10:1566–76

171. Banks LM, Stevenson JC. Modified method of spinal computed tomography for trabecular bone mineral measurements. *J Comput Assist Tomogr* 1986;10:463–7

172. Sandor T, Felsenberg D, Kalender WA, *et al.* Compact and trabecular components of the spine using quantitative computed tomography. *Calcif Tissue Int* 1992;50:502–6

173. Mundinger A, Wiesmeier B, Dinkel E, *et al.* Quantitative image analysis of vertebral body architecture – improved diagnosis in osteoporosis based on high-resolution computed tomography. *Br J Radiol* 1993;66:209–13

174. Wehrli FW, Ford JC, Haddad JG. Osteoporosis: Clinical assessment with quantitative MR imaging in diagnosis. *Radiology* 1995;196:631–41

175. Schick F, Seitz D, Machann J, *et al.* Magnetic resonance bone densitometry. Comparison of different methods based on susceptibility. *Invest Radiol* 1995;30:254–65

176. Spinks TJ. The measurement of calcium and other body elements by *in vivo* neutron activation analysis. In: Stevenson J, ed. *New Techniques in Metabolic Bone Disease.* London: Wright, 1990:157–71

177. Langton CM, Palmer SB, Porter RW. The measurement of broadband ultrasonic attenuation in cancellous bone. *N Engl J Med* 1984;13:89–91

178. Herd RJ, Ramalingham T, Ryan PJ, *et al.* Measurements of broadband ultrasonic attenuation in the calcaneus in premenopausal and postmenopausal women. *Osteoporos Int* 1992;2:247–51

179. Argen M, Karellas A, Leahey D, *et al.* Ultrasound attenuation of the calcaneus: A sensitive and specific discriminator of osteopenia in postmenopausal women. *Calcif Tissue Int* 1991;48:240–4

180. Rossman P, Zagzebski J, Mesina C, *et al.* Comparison of speed of sound and ultrasound attenuation in the os calcis to bone density of the radius, femur and lumbar spine. *Clin Phys Physiol Meas* 1989;10:353–60

181. McCloskey EV, Murray SA, Miller C, *et al.* Broadband ultrasound attenuation in the os calcis:

Relationship to bone mineral at other skeletal sites. *Clin Sci* 1990;78:227–33

182. Baran DT, Kelly AM, Karella A, *et al.* Ultrasound attenuation of the os calcis in women with osteoporosis and hip fractures. *Calcif Tissue Int* 1988;43:138–42

183. Massie A, Reid DM, Porter RW. Screening for osteoporosis: Comparison between dual-energy x-ray absorptiometry and broadband ultrasound attenuation in 1000 perimenopausal women. *Osteoporos Int* 1993;3:107–10

184. Wasnich RD, Ross PD, Hellbrun LK, Vogel JM. Prediction of postmenopausal fracture risk with use of bone mineral measurements. *Am J Obstet Gynecol* 1985;153:745–51

185. Gluer CC, Cummings SR, Bauer DC, *et al.* Osteoporosis: Association of recent fractures with quantitative US findings. *Radiology* 1996;199:725–32

186. Tuppurainen M, Kroger H, Honkanen R, *et al.* Risks of perimenopausal fractures – a prospective population-based study. *Acta Obstet Gynecol Scand* 1995;74:624–8

187. Paganini-Hill A, Ross RK, Gerkins VR, *et al.* Menopausal estrogen therapy and hip fractures. *Ann Intern Med* 1981;95:28–31

188. Weiss NS, Ure BL, Ballard JH, *et al.* Decreased risk of fractures of the hip and lower forearm with postmenopausal use of estrogen. *N Engl J Med* 1980;303:1195–8

189. Hutchinson TA, Polansky SM, Feinstein AR. Postmenopausal oestrogens protect against fractures of the hip and distal radius: A case-controlled study. *Lancet* 1979;ii:705–9

190. Ettinger B, Genant HK, Cann CE. Long term estrogen therapy prevents bone loss and fracture. *Ann Intern Med* 1979;102:319–24

191. Christiansen C, Christensen MS, Larsen N-E, Transbol IB. Pathophysiological mechanisms of estrogen effect on bone metabolism. Dose–response relationships in early postmenopausal women. *J Clin Endocrinol Metab* 1982;55:1124–30

192. Munk-Jensen M, Pors Nielsen S, Obel EB, Bonne Eriksen P. Reversal of postmenopausal vertebral bone loss by oestrogen and progestogen: A double-blind study. *BMJ* 1988;296:1150–2

193. McKay Hart D, Al-Azzawi F, Farish E. Effect of Ossopan alone, oestradiol implants alone or both therapies combined on bone density and bone biochemistry in oophorectomised women. In: Christiansen C, Johansen J, Riis BJ, eds. *Osteoporosis.* Copenhagen: Osteopress, 1987

194. Ryde SJ, Bowen-Simkins K, Bowen-Simkins P, *et al.* The effect of oestradiol implants on regional and total bone mass: A three-year longitudinal study. *Clin Endocrinol* 1994;40:33–8

195. Savvas M, Watson NR, Garnett T, *et al.* Skeletal effects of oral oestrogen compared with subcutaneous oestrogen and testosterone in postmenopausal women. *BMJ* 1988;297:331–3

196. Holland EF, Leather AT, Studd JW. Increase in bone mass of older postmenopausal women with low mineral bone density after one year of percutaneous oestradiol implants. *Br J Obstet Gynaecol* 1995;102:238–42

197. Riis BJ, Thomsen K, Strom V, Christiansen C. The effects of percutaneous estradiol and natural progesterone on postmenopausal bone loss. *Am J Obstet Gynecol* 1987;156:61–5

198. Hillard TC, Whitcroft SJ, Marsh MS, *et al.* Long-term effects of transdermal and oral hormone replacement therapy on postmenopausal bone loss. *Osteoporos Int* 1994;4:341–8

199. Lindsay D, Hart DM, Clark DM. Bone response to termination of oestrogen treatment. *Lancet* 1978; i:1325–7

200. Stevenson JC, Kanis JA, Christiansen C. Bone-density measurement [Letter]. *Lancet* 1992;339:370–1

201. Cauley JA, Seeley DG, Ensrud K, et al., for The Study of Osteoporotic Fractures Research Group. Estrogen replacement therapy and fractures in older women. *Ann Intern Med* 1995;122:9–16

202. Kanis JA. Treatment of osteoporosis in elderly women. *Am J Med* 1995;98:60–6S

203. Kimble RB, Matayoshi A.B, Vannice JL, et al. Simultaneous block of interleukin-1 and tumor necrosis factor is required to completely prevent bone loss in the early postovariectomy period. *Endocrinology* 1995;136:3054–61

204. Vedi S, Crocher PI, Garrahan NJ, Compston JE. Effects of hormone replacement therapy on cancellous bone structure in postmenopausal women. *Bone* 1996;19:69–72

205. Delmas DD, Bjarnason NH, Mitlak BH, et al. Effects of raloxifene on bone mineral density, serum cholesterol concentrations, and uterine endometrium in postmenopausal women. *N Engl J Med* 1997;337:1641–7

206. Ettinger B, Black S, Cummings H, et al., for The MORE Study Group. Raloxifene reduces the risk of incident vertebral fractures: 24-month interim analyses. Abstracts of the European Congress of Osteoporosis. *Osteoporos Int* 1998

207. Gruber HE, Ivey JL, Baylink DJ, et al. Long–term calcitonin therapy in postmenopausal osteoporosis. *Metabolism* 1984;33:295–303

208. MacIntyre I, Stevenson JC, Whitehead MI, et al. Calcitonin for the prevention of postmenopausal bone loss. *Lancet* 1988;ii:1481–3

209. Kollerup G, Hermann AP, Brixen K, et al. Effects of salmon calcitonin suppositories on bone mass and turnover in established osteoporosis. *Calcif Tissue Int* 1994;54:12–15

210. Reginster JY, Jupsin I, Deroisy R, et al. Prevention of postmenopausal bone loss by rectal calcitonin. *Calcif Tissue Int* 1995;56:539–42

211. Overgaard K, Riis BJ, Christiansen C, et al. Nasal calcitonin the treatment of established osteoporosis. *Clin Endocrinol* 1989;30:435–42

212. Reginster JY, Denis D, Albert A, et al. 1-year controlled randomised trial of prevention of early postmenopausal bone loss by intranasal calcitonin. *Lancet* 1987;ii:1481–3

213. Overgaard K. Effect of intranasal salmon calcitonin therapy on bone mass and bone turnover in early postmenopausal women: A dose–response study. *Calcif Tissue Int* 1994;55:82–6

214. Overgaard K, Lindsay R, Christiansen C. Patient responsiveness to calcitonin salmon nasal spray: A subanalysis of a 2-year study. *Clin Ther* 1995;17:680–5

215. Reginster JY, Denis D, Deroisy R, et al. Long-term (3 years) prevention of trabecular postmenopausal bone loss with low-dose intermittent nasal salmon calcitonin. *J Bone Miner Res* 1994;9:69–73

216. Reginster JY, Deroisy R, Lecart MP, et al. A double-blind, placebo-controlled, dose-finding trial of intermittent nasal salmon calcitonin for prevention of postmenopausal lumbar spine bone loss. *Am J Med* 1995;98:452–8

217. Ellerington MC, Hillard TC, Whitcroft SI, et al. Intranasal salmon calcitonin for the prevention and treatment of postmenopausal osteoporosis. *Calcif Tissue Int* 1996;59:6–11

218 Silverman SL, Chesnut C, Andriano K, et al. Salmon calcitonin nasal spray (NS-CT) reduces risk of vertebral fractures (VF) in established osteoporosis and has continuous efficacy with prolonged treatment: accrued 5 year worldwide data of the PROOF Study. *Bone* 1998;23 (Suppl 5):abstr 1108

219. Storm T, Thamsborg G, Sorensen OH, Lund B. The effects of etidronate therapy in postmenopausal osteoporotic women: Preliminary results. In: Christiansen C, Johansen J, Riis BJ, eds. *Osteoporosis*. Viborg: Norhaven Bogtrykken A/S, 1987:1172–6

220. Genant HK, Harris ST, Steiger P, et al. The effects of etidronate therapy in postmenopausal osteoporotic women: Preliminary results. In: Christiansen C, Johansen J, Riis BJ, eds. Osteoporosis. Viborg: Norhaven Bogtrykken A/S, 1987:1177–81

221. Roux C, Oriente P, Laan R, et al. Randomized trial of effect of cyclical etidronate in the prevention of corticosteroid-induced bone loss. J Clin Endocrinol Metab 1998;83:1128–33

222. Valkema R, Papapoulis SE, Vismans F-JFE, et al. A four-year continuous gain in bone mass in APD-treated osteoporosis. In: Christiansen C, Johansen J, Riis BJ, eds. Osteoporosis. Viborg: Norhaven Bogtrykken A/S, 1987:836–9

223. Reid IR, Wattie DJ, Evans MC, et al. Continuous therapy with pamidronate, a potent bisphosphonate, in postmenopausal osteoporosis. J Clin Endocrinol Metab 1994;79:1595–9

224. Lees B, Garland SW, Walton C, et al. Role of oral pamidronate in preventing bone loss in postmenopausal women. Osteoporos Int 1996;6:480–5

225. Liberman UA, Weiss SR, Broll J, et al., for The Alendronate Phase III Osteoporosis Treatment Study Group. Effect of oral alendronate on bone mineral density and the incidence of fractures in postmenopausal osteoporosis. N Engl J Med 1995; 333:1437–43

226. Chesnut CH IIIrd, McClung MR, Ensrud KE, et al. Alendronate treatment of the postmenopausal osteoporotic woman: Effect of multiple dosages on bone mass and bone remodeling. Am J Med 1995; 99:144–52

227. Black DM, Cummings SR, Karpf DB, et al., for The Fracture Intervention Trial Research Group. Randomised trial of effect of alendronate on risk of fracture in women with existing vertebral fractures. Lancet 1996;348:1535–41

228. Beneton MNC, Yates AJP, Rogers S, et al. Stanozolol stimulates remodelling of trabecular bone and the net formation of bone at the endocortical surface. Clin Sci 1991;81:543–9

229. Erdtsieck RJ, Pols HA, van Kuijk C, et al. Course of bone mass during and after hormonal replacement therapy with and without addition of nandrolone decanoate. J Bone Miner Res 1994;9:277–83

230. Guesens P, Dequeker J. Long–term effect of nandrolone decanoate, 1α–hydroxyvitamin D_3 or intermittent calcium infusion therapy on bone mineral content, bone remodeling and fracture rate in symptomatic osteoporosis: A double–blind controlled study. J Bone Miner Res 1986;1:347–57

231. Chesnut CH, Ivey JL, Gruber HE, et al. Stanozolol in postmenopausal osteoporosis: Therapeutic efficacy and possible mechanisms of action. Metabolism 1983;32:571–80

232. Chesnut CH, Nelp WB, Baylink DJ, Denney JD. Effect of methandrostenolone on postmenopausal bone wasting as assessed by changes in total bone mineral mass. Metabolism 1977;26:267–77

233. Aloia JK, Kapoor A, Vaswani A, Cohn SH. Changes in body composition following therapy for osteoporosis with methandrostenolone. Metabolism 1981;30:1076–9

234. Godsland IF, Shennan NM, Wynn V. Insulin action and dynamics modelling in patients taking the anabolic steroid methandienone (Dianabol). Clin Sci 1986;71:665–73

235. Stout RW. Insulin and atheroma: 20-yr perspective. Diabetes Care 1990;13:631–54

236. Mamelle N, Meunier PG, Dusan R, et al. Risk–benefit ratio of sodium fluoride treatment in primary vertebral osteoporosis. Lancet 1988;ii:361–5

237. Riggs BL, Seeman E, Hodgson SF, et al. Effect of the fluoride/calcium regimen on vertebral fracture occurrence in postmenopausal osteoporosis:

Comparison with conventional therapy. *N Engl J Med* 1982;306:446–50

238. Baud CA, Very JM, Courvoisier B. Biophysical studies of bone mineral in biopsies of osteoporotic patients before and after long-term treatment with fluoride. *Bone* 1988;9:361–5

239. Pak CY, Sakhaee K, Adams-Huet B, *et al.* Treatment of postmenopausal osteoporosis with slow-release sodium fluoride. Final report of a randomized controlled trial. *Ann Intern Med* 1995;123:401–8

240. Hedlund IR, Gallagher JC. Increased incidence of hip fracture in women treated with sodium fluoride. *J Bone Miner Res* 1989;4:223–5

241. Frost HM. Treatment of osteoporosis by manipulation of coherent bone cell populations. *Clin Orth Rel Res* 1979;143:227–44

242. Rasmussen H, Bordier P, Marie P, *et al.* Effect of combined therapy with phosphate and calcitonin on bone volume in osteoporosis. *Metab Bone Dis Rel Res* 1980;2:107–11

243. Marie PJ, Caulin F. Mechanisms underlying the effects of phosphate and calcitonin on bone histology in postmenopausal osteoporosis. *Bone* 1986;7:17–22

244. Hasling C, Charles P, Jensen FT, Mosekilde L. A comparison of the effects of oestrogen/progestogen, high-dose oral calcium, intermittent cyclic etidronate and an ADFR regime on calcium kinetics and bone mass in postmenopausal women with spinal osteoporosis. *Osteoporos Int* 1994;4:191–203

245. Hesch R-D, Busch U, Prokop M, *et al.* Increase of vertebral bone density by combination therapy with pulsatile 1–38hPTH and sequential addition of calcium nasal spray in osteoporotic patients. *Calcif Tissue Int* 1989;44:176–80

246. Lindsay R, Nieves J, Formica C, *et al.* Randomised controlled study of effect of parathyroid hormone on vertebral-bone mass and fracture incidence among postmenopausal women on oestrogen with osteoporosis. *Lancet* 1997;350:550–5

247. Ott SM, Chesnut CH. Calcitriol treatment is not effective in postmenopausal osteoporosis. *Ann Intern Med* 1989;110:267–74

248. Nordin BEC, Horsman A, Crilly RG, *et al.* Treatment of spinal osteoporosis in postmenopausal women. *BMJ* 1980;280:451–4

249. Hansen MA. Assessment of age and risk factors on bone density and bone turnover in healthy premenopausal women. *Osteoporos Int* 1994;4:123–8

250. Chapuy MC, Chapuy P, Thomas JL, *et al.* Biochemical effects of calcium and vitamin D supplementation in elderly, institutionalized, vitamin D-deficient patients. *Rev Rhum Mal Osteoartic* (English edn) 1996;63:135–40

251. Dawson-Hughes B, Harris SS, Krall EA, *et al.* ates of bone loss in postmenopausal women randomly assigned to one of two dosages of vitamin D. *Am J Clin Nutr* 1995;61:1140–5

252. Dawson-Hughes B, Dallal GE, Krall EA, *et al.* A controlled trial of the effect of calcium supplementation on bone density in postmenopausal women. *N Engl J Med* 1990;323:878–83

253. Reid IR, Ames RW, Evans MC, *et al.* Long-term effects of calcium supplementation on bone loss and fractures in postmenopausal women: A randomized controlled trial. *Am J Med* 1995;98:331–5

254. Heaney RP. The role of nutrition in prevention and management of osteoporosis. *Clin Obstet Gynecol* 1987;50:833–46

255. Chow R, Harrison JE, Notarius C. Effects of two randomised exercise programmes on bone mass of healthy postmenopausal women. *BMJ* 1987;295:1441–4

256. Lohman T, Going S, Pamenter R, et al. Effects of resistance training on regional and total bone mineral density in premenopausal women: A randomized prospective study. J Bone Miner Res 1995;10:1015–24

257. Greendale GA, Barrett-Connor E, Edelstein S, et al. Lifetime leisure exercise and osteoporosis. The Rancho Bernardo study. Am J Epidemiol 1995;14:951–9

258. Dalsky GP, Stocke KS, Ehsani AA, et al. Weight-bearing exercise training and lumbar bone mineral content in postmenopausal women. Ann Intern Med 1988;108:824–8

259. Prudham D, Evans JG. Factors associated wth falls in the elderly: A community study. Age Ageing 1981;10:141–6

260. Tinnetti ME, Speechley M, Ginter SF. Risk factors for falls among elderly persons living in the community. N Engl J Med 1988;319:1701–7

261. Lauritzen JB, Petersen MM, Lund B. Effect of external hip protectors on hip fractures. Lancet 1993;341:11–13

262. Citron JT, Ettinger B, Genant HK. Prediction of peak premenopausal bone mass using a scale of weighted variables. In: Christiansen C, Johansen J, Riis BJ, ed. Osteoporosis. Kobenhavn: Osteopress, 1987:146–9

263. Yano K, Wasnich RD, Vogel JM, Heilbrun LK. Bone mineral measurements among middle-aged and elderly Japanese residents in Hawaii. Am J Epidemiol 1984;119:751–64

264. Sowers MR, Wallace RD, Lemke JH. Correlates of mid-radius bone density among postmenopausal women: A community study. Am J Clin Nutr 1985;41:1045–53

265. Kroger H, Tuppurainen M, Honkanen R, et al. Bone mineral density and risk factors for osteoporosis – a population-based study of 1600 perimenopausal women. Calcif Tissue Int 1994;55:1–7

266. Bauer DC, Browner WS, Cauley JA, et al. for The Study of Osteoporosis Fractures Research Group. Factors associated with appendicular bone mass in older women. Ann Intern Med 1993;118:657–65

267. Wasnich RD, Ross PD, Vogel JM, Maclean CJ. The relative strengths of osteoporotic risk factors in a prospective study of postmenopausal osteoporosis. J Bone Miner Res 1987;2(Suppl 1):343

268. Ravnikar A. Compliance with hormone therapy. Am J Obstet Gynecol 1987;156:1332–4

269. Wallace WA, Price VA, Elliot CA, et al. Hormone replacement therapy: Acceptability to Nottingham postmenopausal women with a risk factor for osteoporosis. J R Soc Med 1990;83:699–701

270. Hunt K. Perceived value of treatment among a group of long-term users of hormone replacement therapy. J R Coll Gen Pract 1988;38:398–401

271. Bush TL, Barrett-Connor E, Cowan LD, et al. Cardiovascular mortality and non-contraceptive use of estrogen in women: Results from the Lipid Research Clinics Program Follow–Up Study. Circulation 1987;75:1102–9

272. Paganini-Hill A, Ross RK, Henderson BE. Postmenopausal oestrogen therapy and stroke: A prospective study. BMJ 1988;297:519–22

Section 2 Osteoporosis Illustrated

List of illustrations

Figure 1.1
Graph showing incidence rates for the three most common osteoporotic fractures

Figure 1.2
Graph showing hip fracture incidence world-wide

Figure 1.3
Graph showing relationship of bone density to fracture

Figure 1.4
Graph showing correlation between vertebral and forearm trabecular bone density

Figure 2.1
Histology showing normal iliac crest bone density

Figure 2.2
Photomicrograph of cortical bone

Figure 2.3
SEM of a layer or 'pavement' of osteoblasts

Figure 2.4
Histology of osteoblasts and multinucleated osteoclasts

Figure 2.5
SEM of osteoclasts *in vitro*

Figure 2.6
SEM of osteoclastic bone resorption *in vitro*

Figure 2.7
SEM of osteocytes in bone lacunae

Figure 2.8
SEM showing osteocytes and their canalicular processes

Figure 2.9
SEM of collagen fibers in lamellar bone matrix

Figure 2.10
Graphic representation of the developing and mature cells of bone

Figure 2.11
SEM showing active osteoclastic bone resorption

Figure 2.12
Histology showing a resorption lacune in trabecular bone

Figure 2.13
SEMs showing evolving Haversian system in the bone cortex

Figure 2.14
Back-scattered EM showing stages of bone remodeling

Figure 2.15
Biopsy sections of iliac crest showing remodeling cycle in trabecular bone

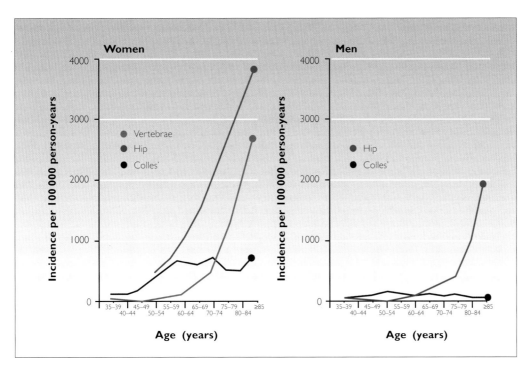

Figure 1.1 Incidence rates for the three most common osteoporotic fractures, plotted as a function of age at time of fracture. Rates are much lower in men and occur at a later age than in women. From reference 14, with permission

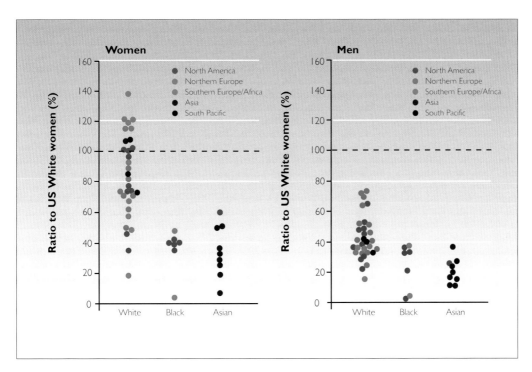

Figure 1.2 Hip fracture incidence around the world expressed as a ratio of the rates observed to those expected in the US for white women of the same age. From reference 3, with permission

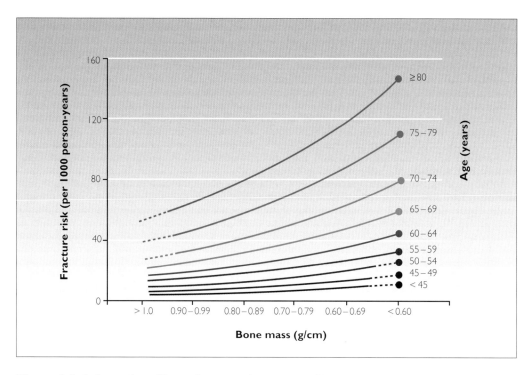

Figure 1.3 Relationship of bone density to fracture at different ages allows prediction of future fracture risk. From reference 21, with permission

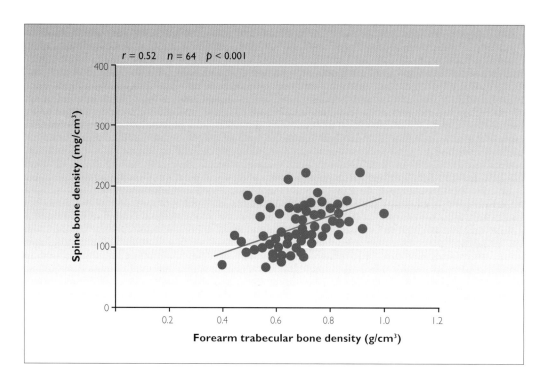

Figure 1.4 Correlation between vertebral and forearm trabecular bone density as measured by quantitative computed tomography (QCT). The relationship is highly significant, but not predictive. From reference 121, with permission

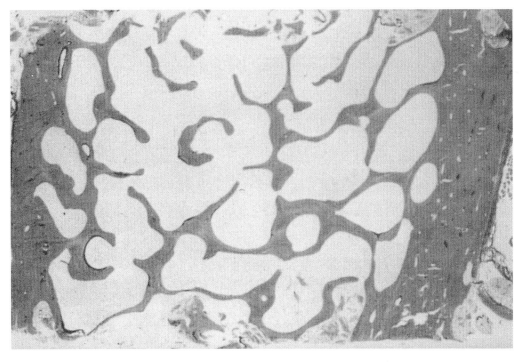

Figure 2.1 Normal iliac crest bone (Goldner's tri-chrome stain) showing inner and outer cortices and intervening trabecular bone. From Dempster DW, Shane E. *Principles and Practice of Endocrinology and Metabolism*. Philadelphia: JB Lippincott Co., 1990:475–80, with permission

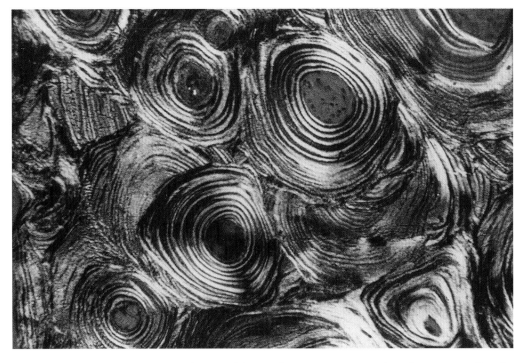

Figure 2.2 Photomicrograph of cortical bone showing concentric lamellae surrounding the central Haversian canal. From Coe F, Favus MJ, eds. *Disorders of Bone and Mineral Metabolism*. New York: Raven Press, 1992, with permission

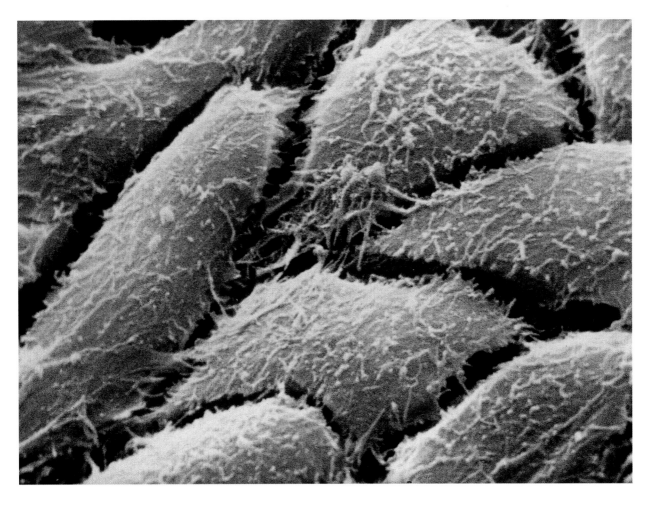

Figure 2.3 Scanning electron micrograph (SEM) of a layer or 'pavement' of osteoblasts. Courtesy of Professor Sheila Jones

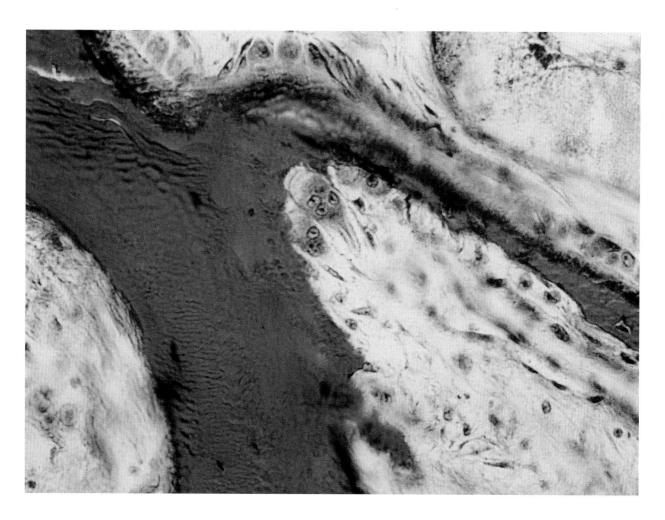

Figure 2.4 Histology showing osteoblasts on one side of a trabecular structure with multi-nucleated osteoclasts on the other. Osteoblasts are polarized, mononuclear, fusiform to cuboidal cells with basophilic cytoplasm. They form bone matrix (osteoid) which mineralizes in a two-phase process to mature bone. Courtesy of Dr Flemming Melsen

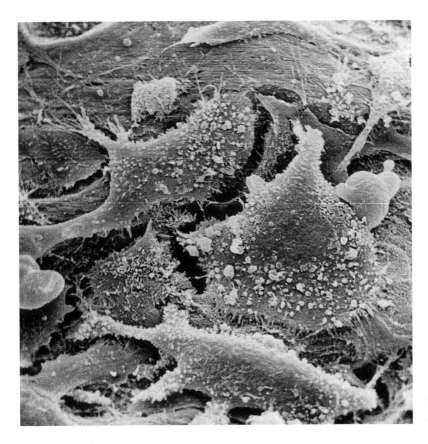

Figure 2.5 SEM of osteoclasts *in vitro*. Courtesy of Professor Alan Boyde

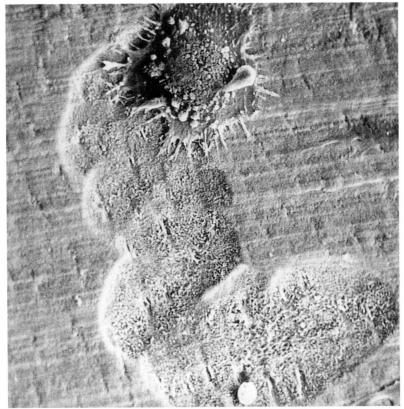

Figure 2.6 SEM showing osteoclastic resorption of bone *in vitro*. Courtesy of Professor Alan Boyde

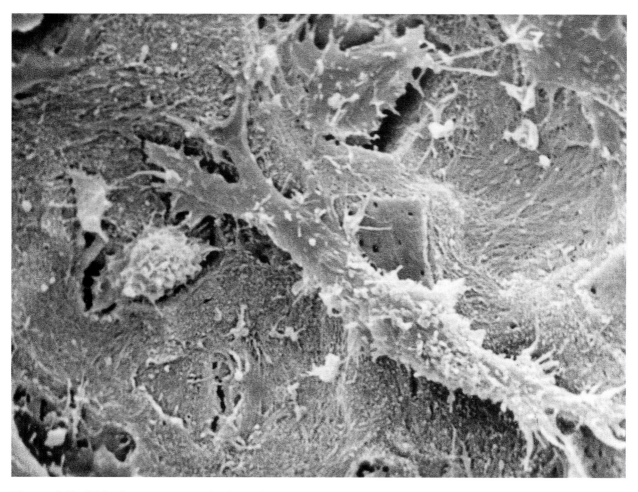

Figure 2.7 SEM of osteocytes in the bone lacunae. A 'liberated' osteocyte is seen on the surface. Courtesy of Professor Alan Boyde

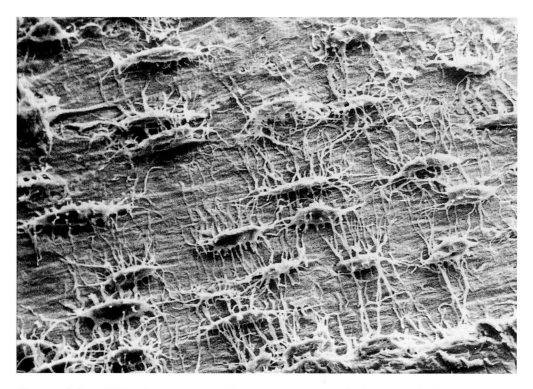

Figure 2.8 SEM of a cast to show osteocytes and their canalicular processes. Courtesy of Professor Alan Boyde

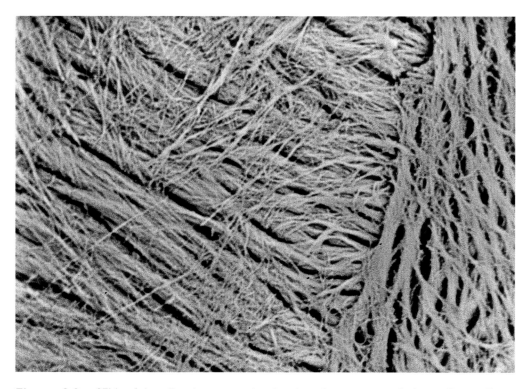

Figure 2.9 SEM of lamellar bone matrix showing the pattern of the collagen fibers. Courtesy of Professor Alan Boyde

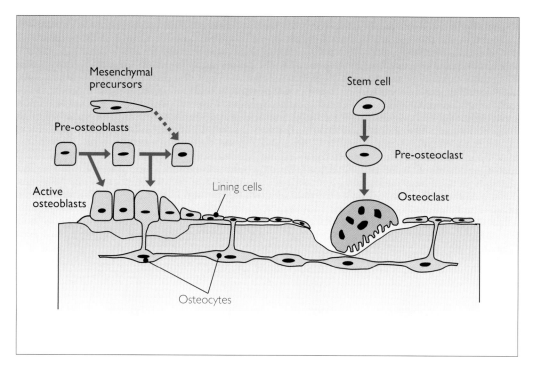

Figure 2.10 Diagrammatic representation of the developing and mature cells of bone to show the relationship between osteocytes and surface cells. From Stevenson JC, Lindsay RL, *Osteoporosis.* London: Chapman & Hall, with permission

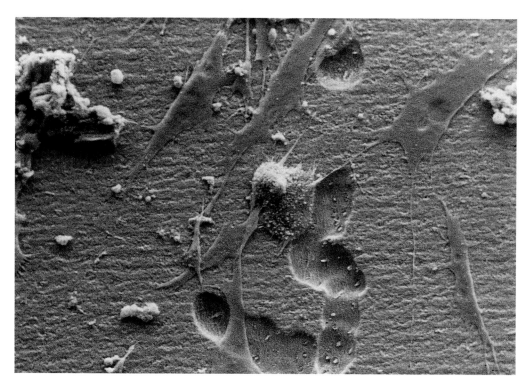

Figure 2.11 SEM from a time-lapse video of osteoclastic bone resorption showing a track of resorption pits. Courtesy of Professor Alan Boyde

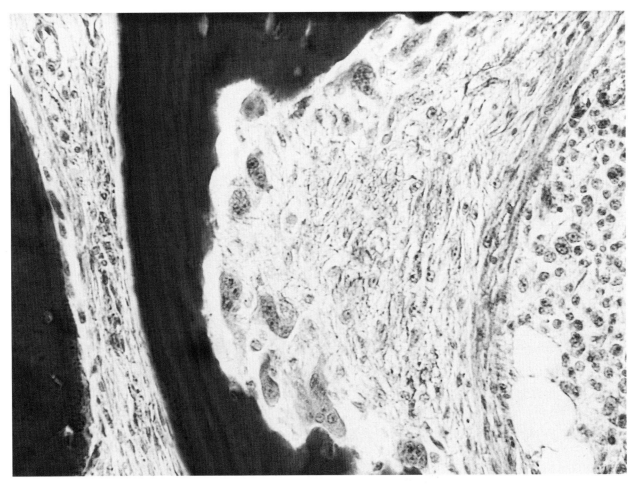

Figure 2.12 Histology from a patient with primary hyperparathyroidism showing a resorption lacune in trabecular bone (Howship's lacune) with multinucleated osteoclasts. Osteoclastic bone resorption includes bone matrix as well as bone mineral. The final depth of the resorption lacune, which reflects the amount of activity of the osteoclasts, is measured by counting the number of missing lamellae. Courtesy of Dr Flemming Melsen

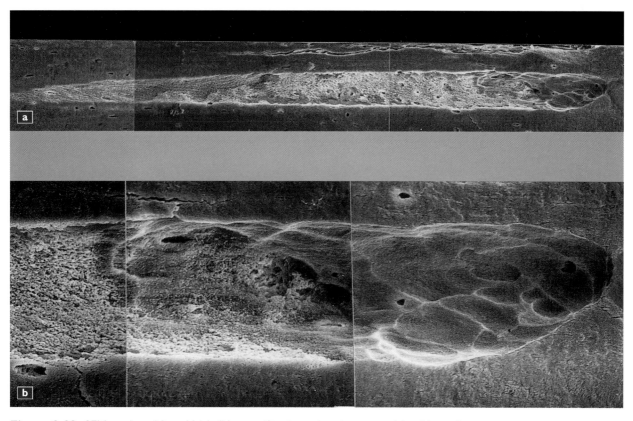

Figure 2.13 SEMs at low (a) and high (b) magnifications showing an evolving Haversian system in the bone cortex (viewed longitudinally). The cutting zone (to the right) is followed by the reversal zone and the mineralization front, with new bone then closing the canal. From Coe F, Favus MJ, eds. *Disorders of Bone and Mineral Metabolism*. New York: Raven Press, 1992, with permission

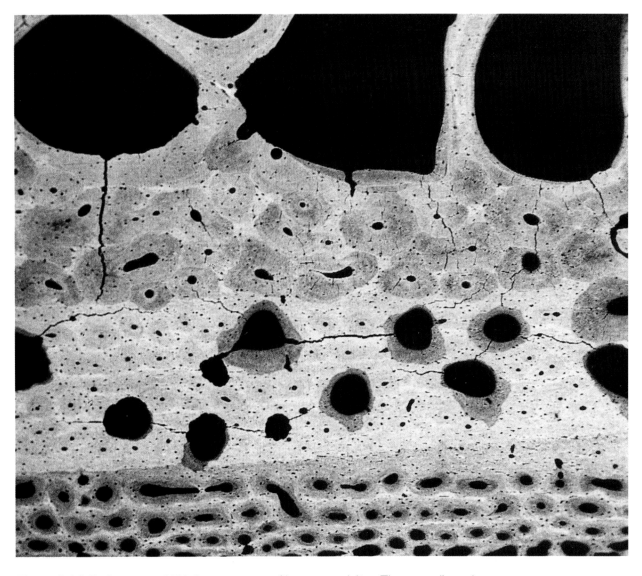

Figure 2.14 Back-scattered EM showing stages of bone remodeling. The outer (lower) cortex shows predominantly resorption and many Haversian canals whereas the inner (upper) cortex near the trabecular surface shows new bone formation closing the canals. There is a mixed pattern in the central cortical area. Courtesy of Professor Alan Boyde

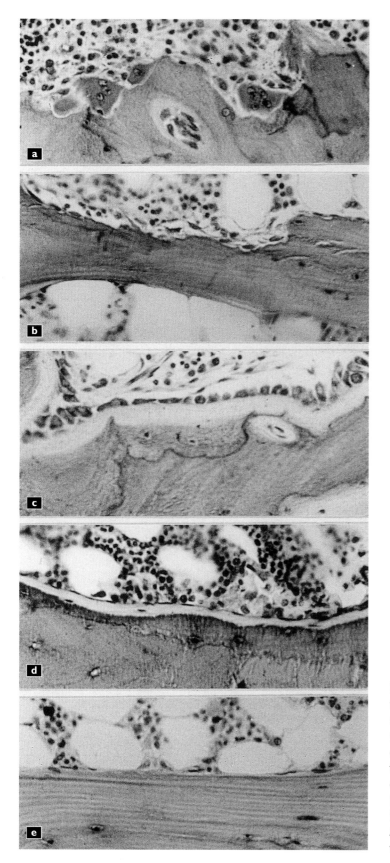

Figure 2.15 Histological biopsy sections from the iliac crest show the principal phases of the remodeling cycle in trabecular bone: resorption by osteoclasts (a); reversal, with disappearance of the osteoclasts (b); formation, with deposition of osteoid by osteoblasts (c); mineralization of the osteoid (d); and completion of the cycle (e). From Coe F, Favus MJ, eds. *Disorders of Bone and Mineral Metabolism*. New York: Raven Press, 1992, with permission

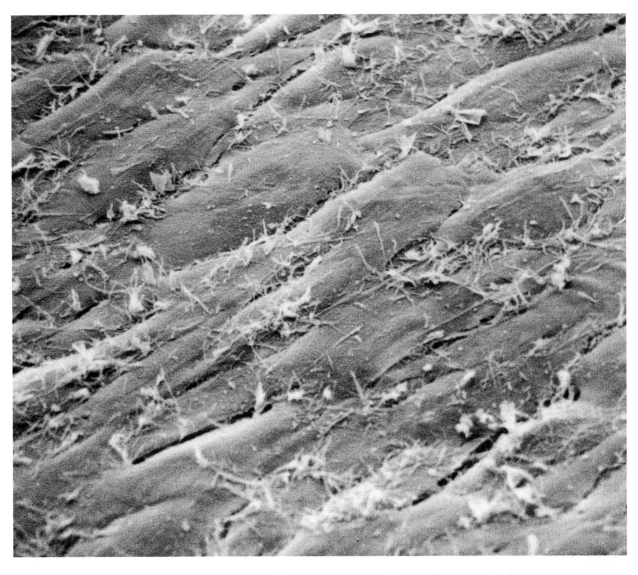

Figure 2.16 SEM of the effects of parathyroid hormone on osteoblasts. There is initial separation followed by spreading and elongation of the cells, which become multilayered. Withdrawal of parathyroid hormone leads to an increase in cell mitosis[52]. Courtesy of Professor Sheila Jones

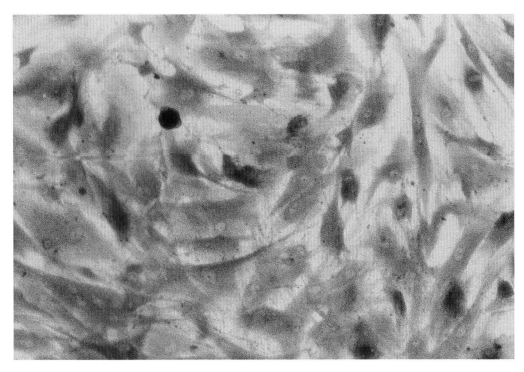

Figure 2.17 Cytoplasmic staining for estradiol receptor-related protein (p29 antigen) results in intense staining of primary human trabecular osteoblast-like cells. From reference 57, with permission

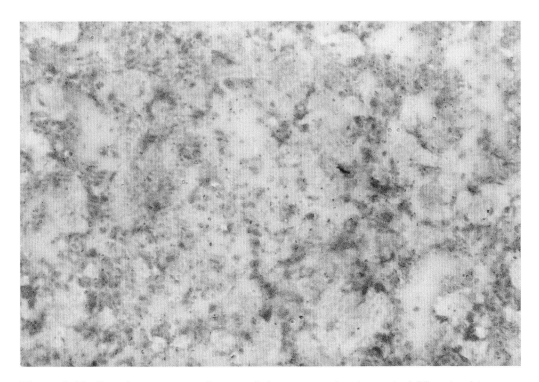

Figure 2.18 Cytoplasmic staining for estradiol receptor-related protein (p29 antigen) in human giant cell tumor imprint. Osteoclasts are clearly visible because of their lack of staining. From reference 57, with permission

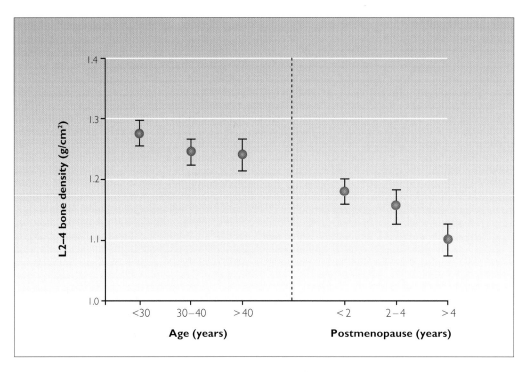

Figure 3.1 Bone density in the lumbar spine (L2–4) in 107 premenopausal and 166 postmenopausal healthy women according to age or time since menopause. There is rapid loss of bone density following the menopause. From reference 85, with permission

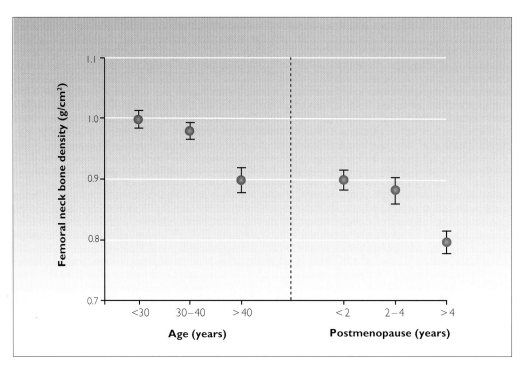

Figure 3.2 Bone density in the femoral neck in 108 premenopausal and 171 postmenopausal healthy women according to age or time since menopause. There is some premenopausal loss of bone density, but more rapid loss following the menopause. From reference 85, with permission

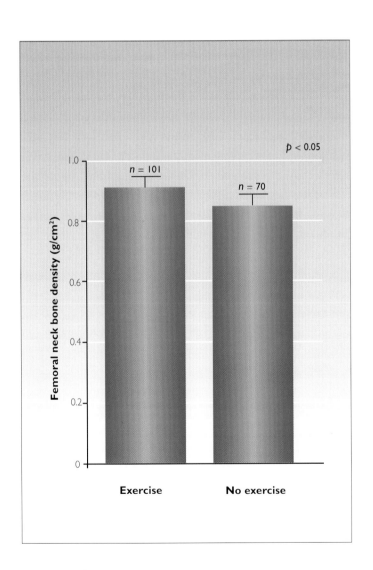

Figure 3.3 Difference in femoral neck bone density between 101 healthy postmenopausal women who took regular weight-bearing exercise and 70 who did not. From Stevenson JC *et al. Osteoporosis.* London: Royal College of Physicians, 1990:119–24, with permission

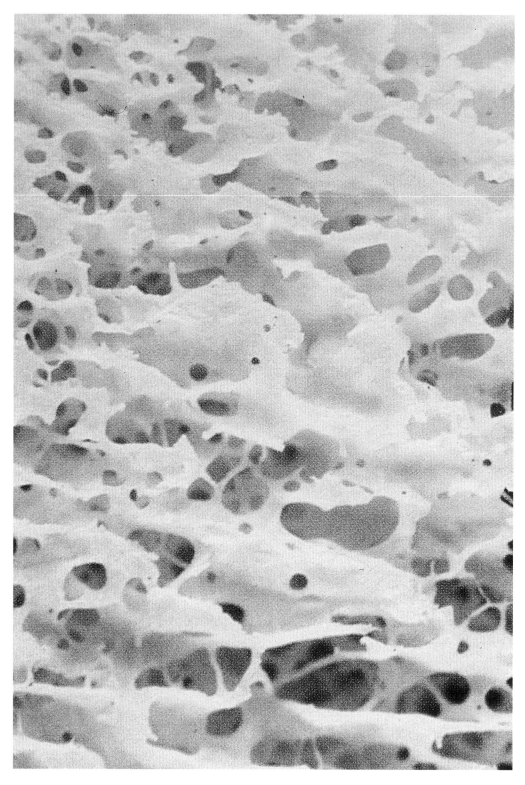

Figure 3.4 Typical isotropic trabecular (or cancellous) bone from a non-weight-bearing part of the skeleton (iliac crest). The tissue forms a three-dimensional lattice of anastomosing plates and struts without a fixed orientation in space. This structure provides the maximum support with a minimum of material. Courtesy of Dr Leif Mosekilde

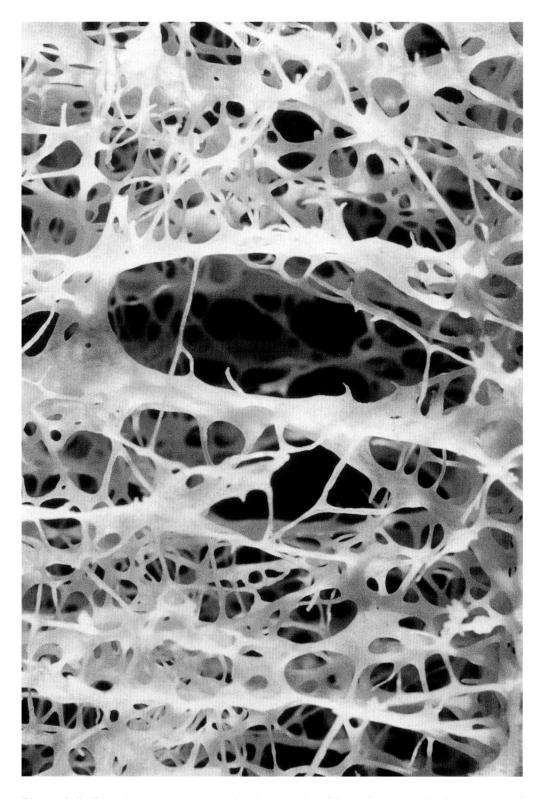

Figure 3.5 Typical anisotropic trabecular (or cancellous) bone from a weight-bearing part of the skeleton (spine). The tissue forms a three-dimensional lattice of thick anastomosing columns and thinner horizontal struts. Courtesy of Dr Leif Mosekilde

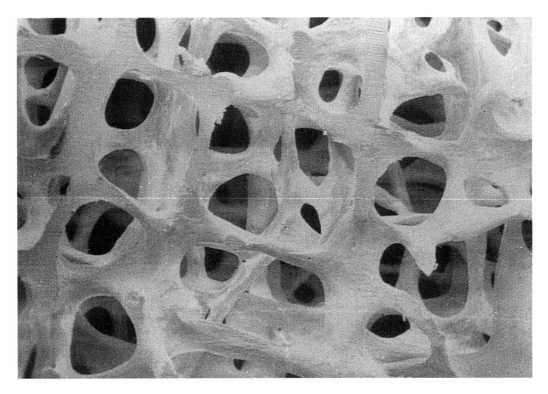

Figure 3.6 SEM of normal trabecular bone showing thick trabecular plates, which are all interconnected. Courtesy of Professor Alan Boyde

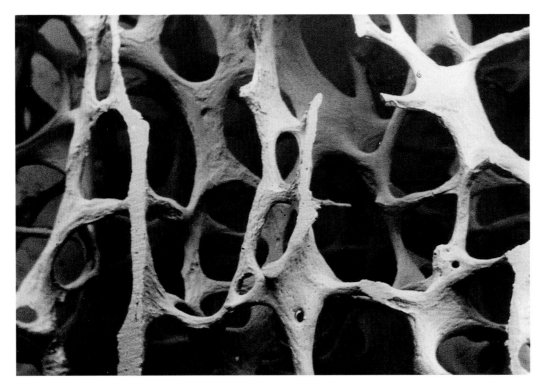

Figure 3.7 SEM of osteoporotic trabecular bone showing marked thinning and disconnection of trabeculae. Courtesy of Professor Alan Boyde

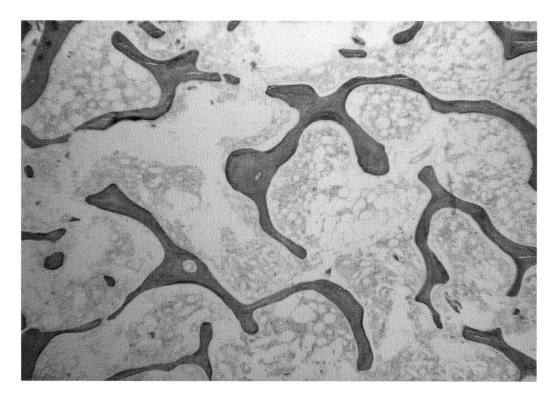

Figure 3.8 Histological biopsy section of iliac crest bone (Goldner's trichrome) from a non-osteoporotic subject shows connectivity of the trabecular elements. Courtesy of Dr David Dempster

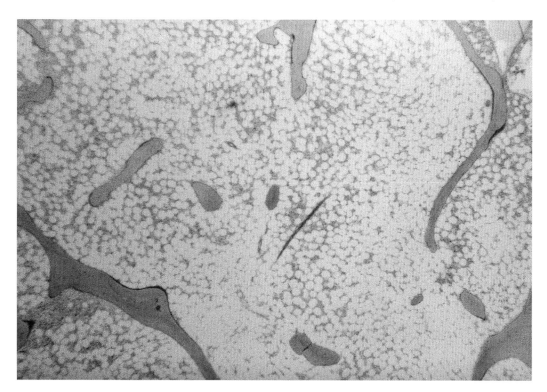

Figure 3.9 Histological biopsy section of iliac crest bone (Goldner's trichrome) from a patient with osteoporosis shows marked loss of trabecular elements. Courtesy of Dr David Dempster

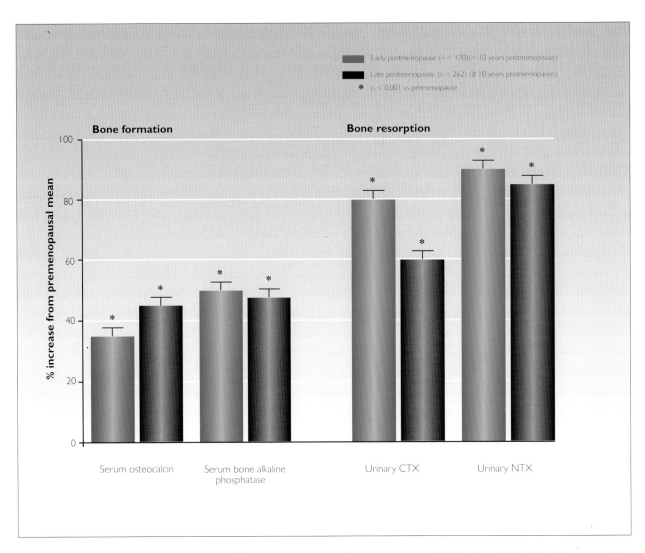

Figure 4.1 Levels of bone formation and bone resorption markers are increased in both early (within 10 years of the menopause; mean 5 years) and late (10 years or more postmenopause; mean 20 years; range 10–40 years) postmenopausal women ($n = 432$). For each marker in each group, mean levels are expressed as a percentage increase ($\pm$ SEM) over the mean of 134 premenopausal women (ages 31–57 years). Both bone formation and resorption were markedly increased at the time of menopause, and a high bone turnover is maintained in late postmenopausal women and in the elderly. NTX, type I cross-linked N telopeptides; CTX, type I C telopeptide breakdown products. Adapted from Garnero et al., J Bone Miner Res 1996;11:337–49, with permission

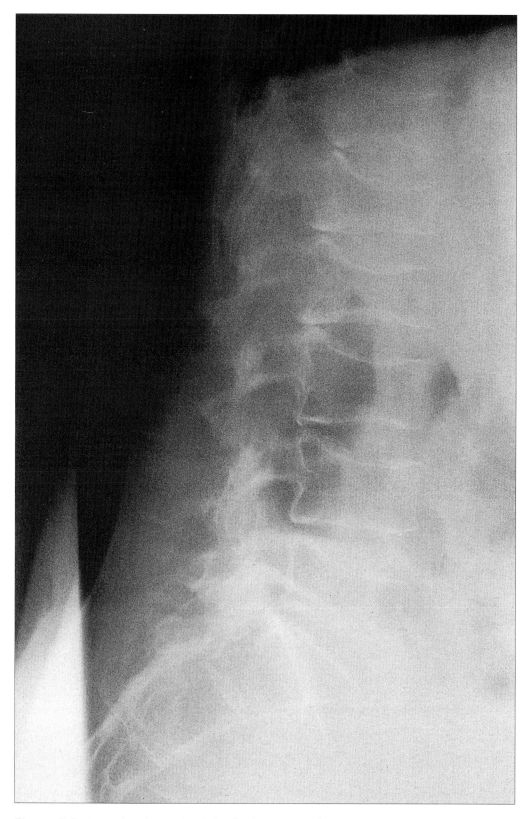

Figure 5.1   Lateral radiograph of the lumbar spine of a patient with osteoporosis shows wedging and compression of several vertebrae. Courtesy of Ms Linda Banks

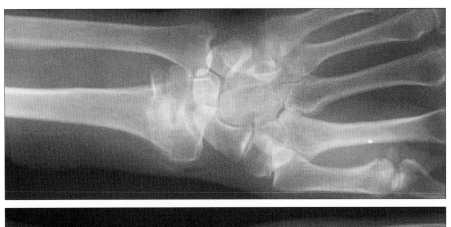

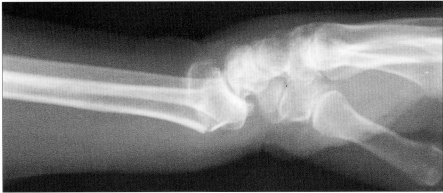

Figure 5.2 Radiographs of the distal forearm showing a Colles' fracture. Courtesy of Mr Paul Allen

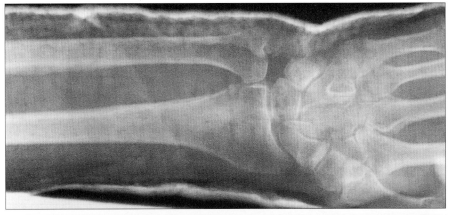

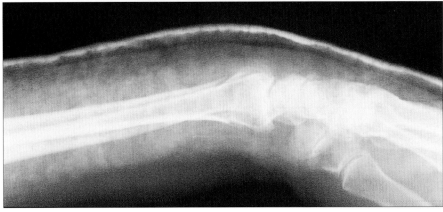

Figure 5.3 Radiographs of the distal forearm showing a Colles' fracture after reduction and external fixation. Courtesy of Mr Paul Allen

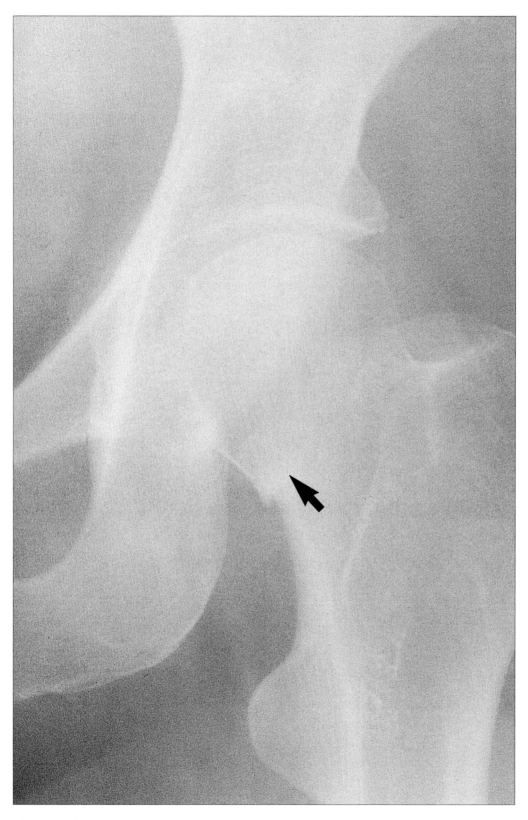

Figure 5.4 Radiograph of the proximal femur showing an intracapsular hip fracture. Courtesy of Mr Paul Allen

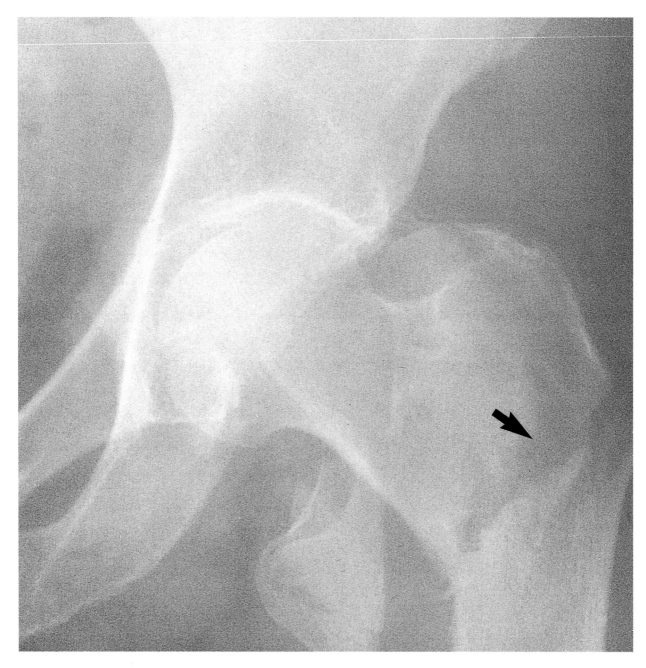

Figure 5.5 Radiograph of the proximal femur showing an extracapsular hip fracture. Courtesy of Mr Paul Allen

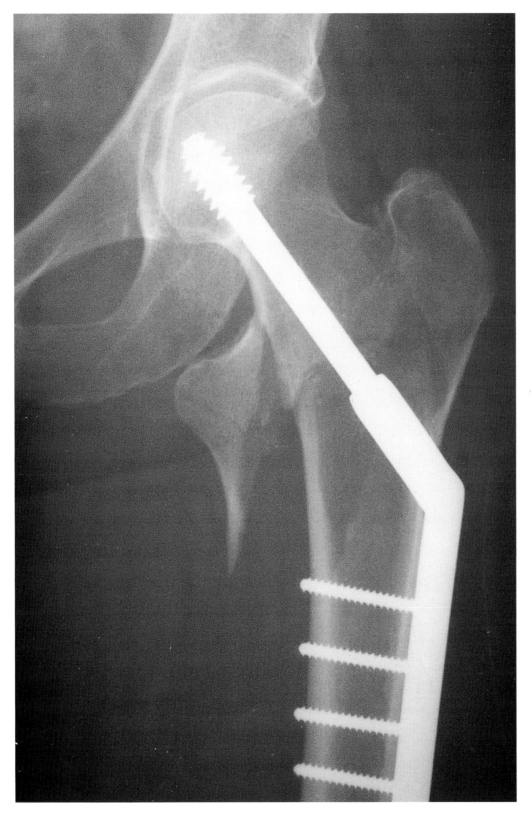

Figure 5.6 Radiograph of the proximal femur showing an extracapsular hip fracture after reduction and internal fixation. Courtesy of Mr Paul Allen

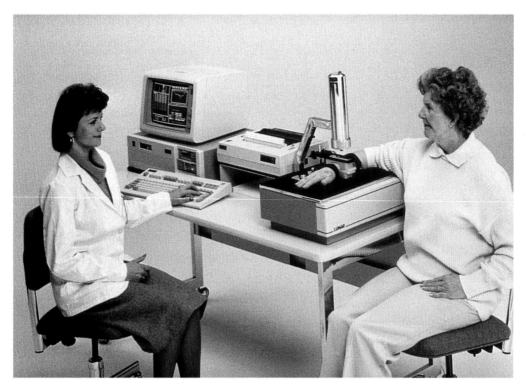

Figure 5.7 Single-photon absorptiometer (SPA; Lunar SP2). Courtesy of Lunar, Madison, WI

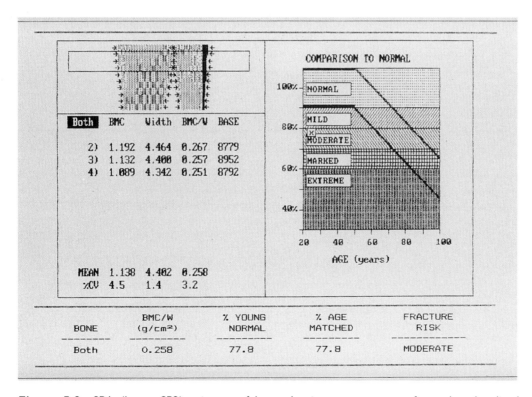

Figure 5.8 SPA (Lunar SP2) printout of bone density measurements from the ultradistal forearm of a young patient with osteoporosis. Courtesy of Lunar, Madison, WI

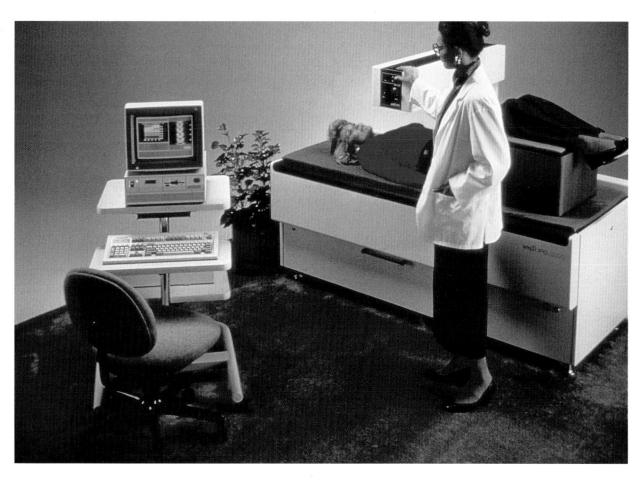

Figure 5.9 Dual-energy X-ray absorptiometer (DEXA; Lunar DPX-IQ). Courtesy of Lunar, Madison, WI

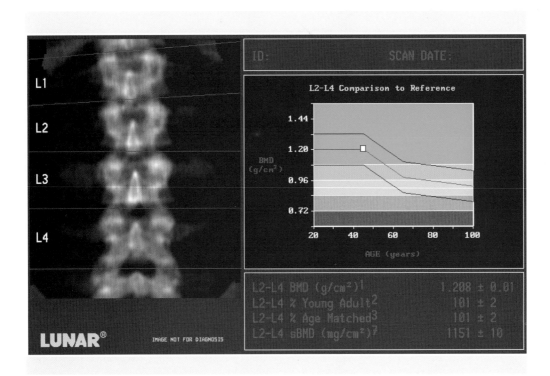

Figure 5.10 DEXA (Lunar DPX-IQ) measurements of lumbar spine bone density in a normal woman (AP view). Courtesy of Lunar, Madison, WI

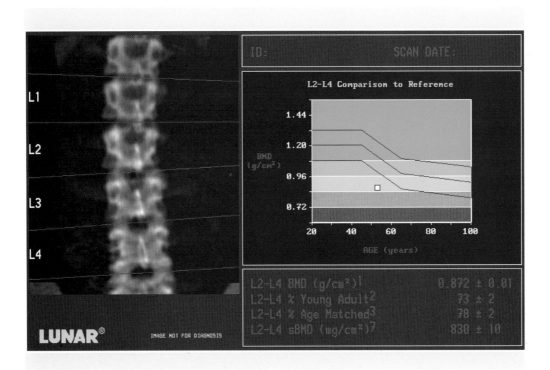

Figure 5.11 DEXA (Lunar DPX-IQ) measurements of lumbar spine bone density in an osteoporotic woman (AP view). Courtesy of Lunar, Madison, WI

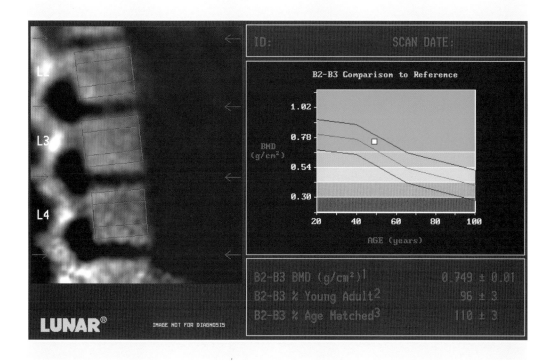

Figure 5.12 DEXA (Lunar DPX-IQ) measurements of lumbar spine bone density in a normal woman (lateral view). Courtesy of Lunar, Madison, WI

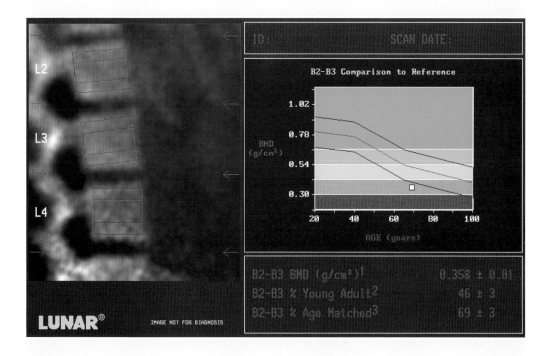

Figure 5.13 DEXA (Lunar DPX-IQ) measurements of lumbar spine bone density in an osteoporotic woman (lateral view). Courtesy of Lunar, Madison, WI

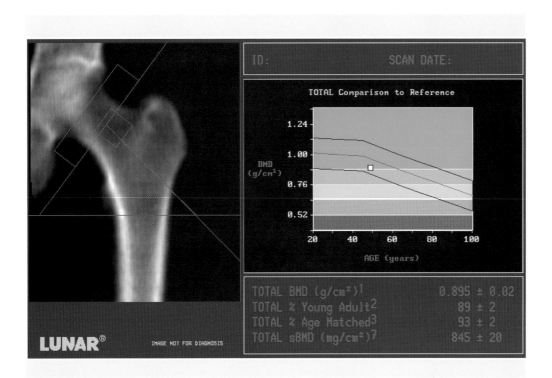

Figure 5.14 DEXA (Lunar DPX-IQ) measurements of femoral neck bone density in a normal woman (AP view). Courtesy of Lunar, Madison, WI

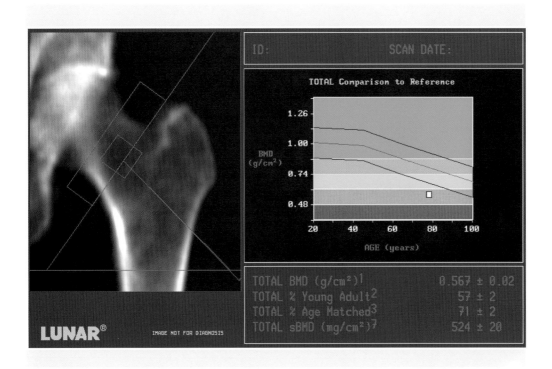

Figure 5.15 DEXA (Lunar DPX-IQ) measurements of femoral neck bone density in an osteoporotic woman (AP view). Courtesy of Lunar, Madison, WI

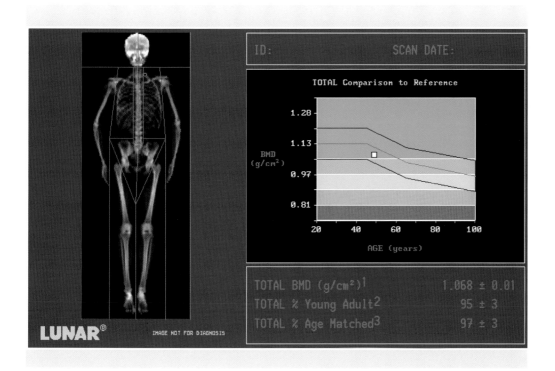

Figure 5.16 DEXA (Lunar DPX-IQ) measurements of total body bone mineral density in a normal woman (AP view). Courtesy of Lunar, Madison, WI

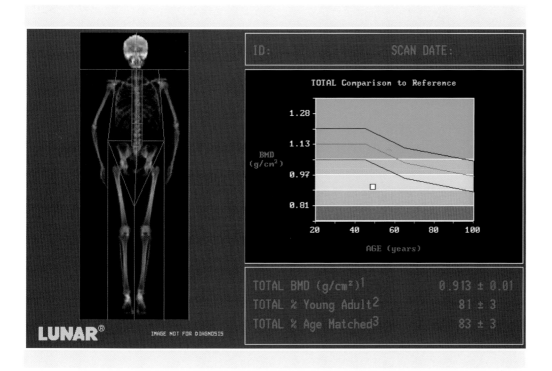

Figure 5.17 DEXA (Lunar DPX-IQ) measurements of total body bone mineral density in an osteoporotic woman (AP view). Courtesy of Lunar, Madison, WI

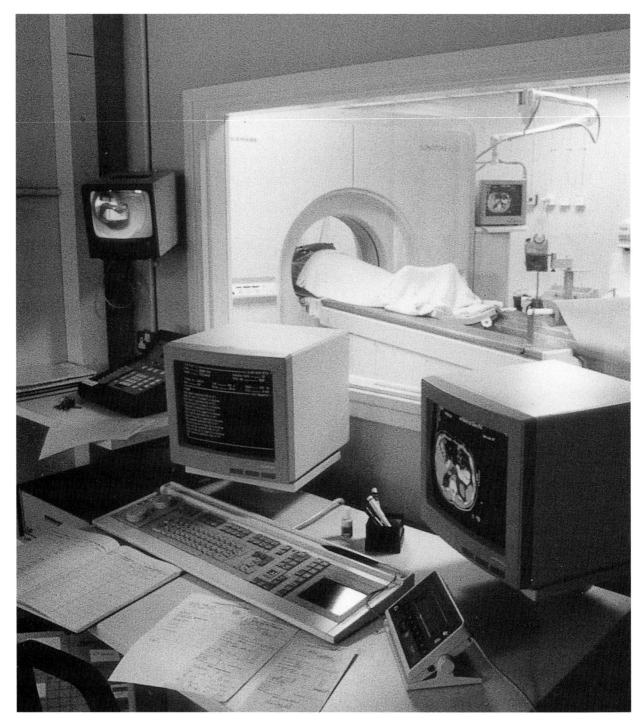

Figure 5.18 Computed tomography (CT) scanner (Siemens Somatom Plus). Courtesy of Ms Linda Banks

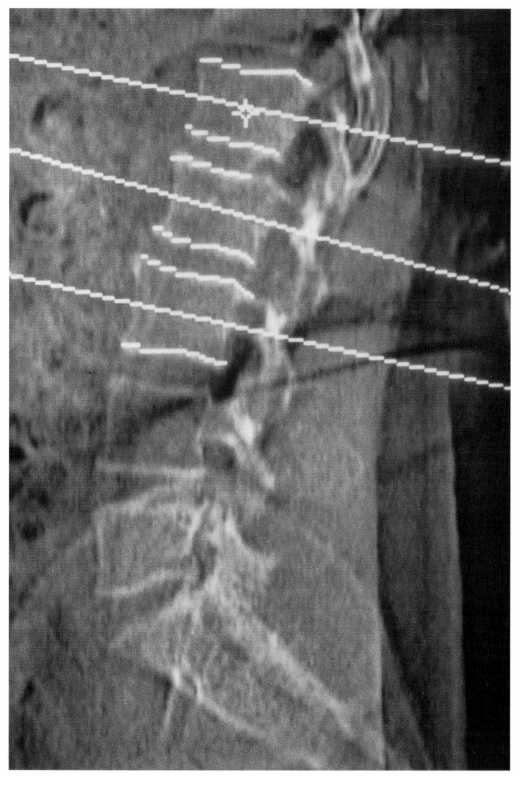

Figure 5.19 Lateral quantitative CT (QCT; Siemens Somatom Plus 2) showing midpoint identification of L1–L3 vertebrae. The patient was scanned on the San Francisco (liquid) calibration phantom. Courtesy of Ms Linda Banks

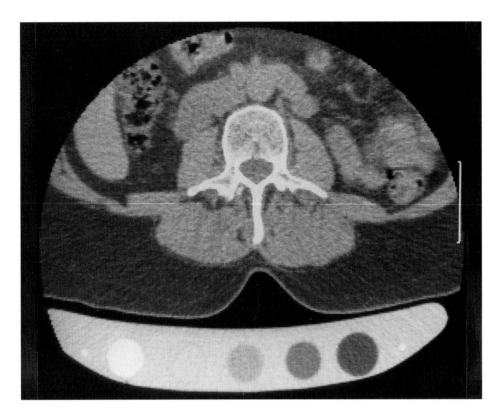

Figure 5.20 Transverse QCT (Siemens Somatom Plus 2) at the midpoint (same patient as in Figure 5.19) shows clear differentiation of cortical from trabecular bone. Courtesy of Ms Linda Banks

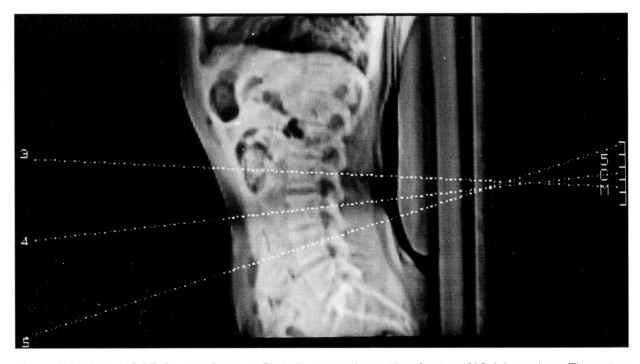

Figure 5.21 Lateral QCT (Siemens Somatom Plus) showing midpoint identification of L2–L4 vertebrae. The patient was scanned on the Siemens (solid) calibration phantom. Courtesy of Ms Linda Banks

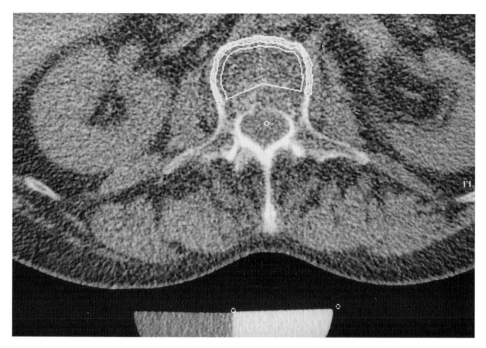

Figure 5.22 Transverse QCT (Siemens Somatom Plus) at the midpoint (same patient as in Figure 5.21) shows clear differentiation of cortical from trabecular bone. Courtesy of Ms Linda Banks

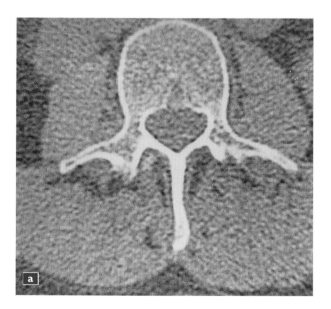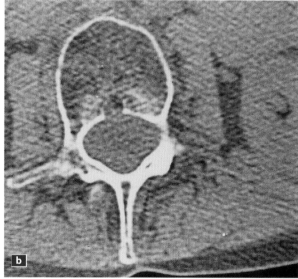

Figure 5.23 Transverse QCTs (Siemens Somatom Plus 2) of lumbar vertebrae in a normal subject (a) and a patient with osteoporosis (b). The clear distinction between outer cortical and inner trabecular bone enables measurement of each component. Courtesy of Ms Linda Banks

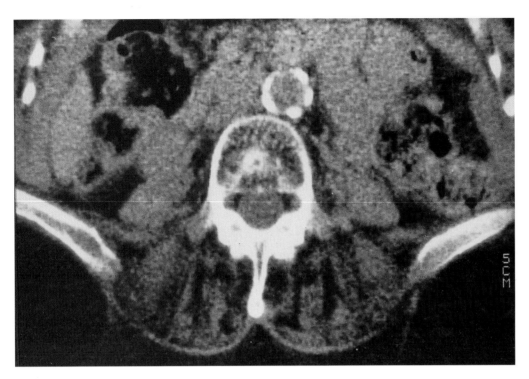

Figure 5.24 Transverse QCT (Siemens Somatom Plus) showing aortic calcification and an intra-vertebral sclerotic area, both of which affect DPA and DEXA measurements. Courtesy of Ms Linda Banks

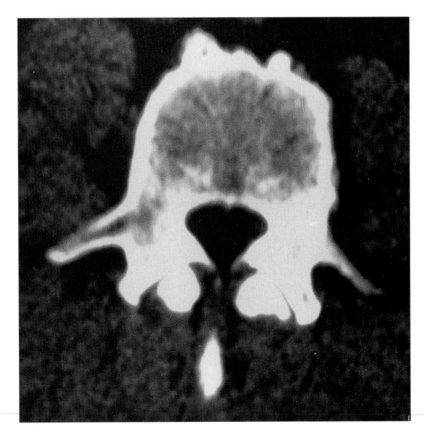

Figure 5.25 Transverse QCT (Siemens Somatom Plus) showing extraneous calcification in the vertebral cortex due to degenerative changes which affects DPA and DEXA measurements. Courtesy of Ms Linda Banks

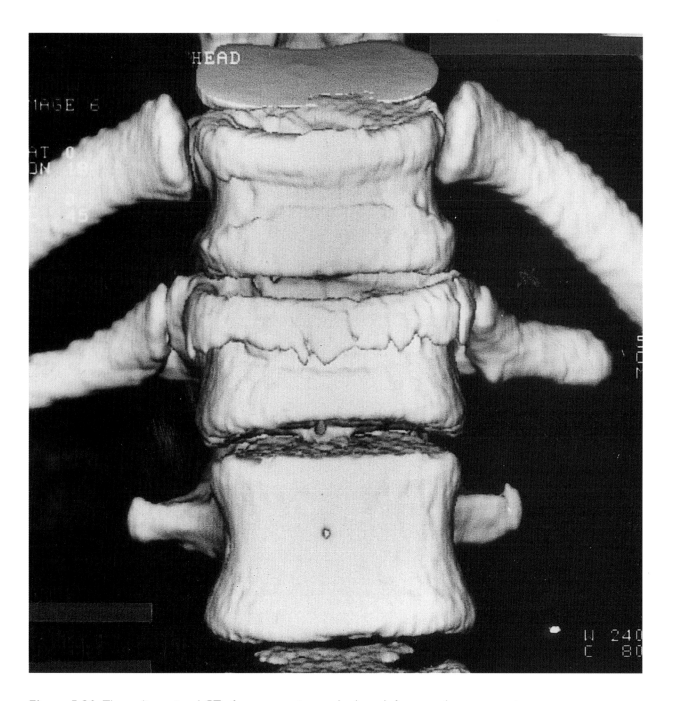

Figure 5.26 Three-dimensional CT of osteoporotic vertebral crush fractures (anteroposterior view). Courtesy of Siemens AG, Erlangen, Germany

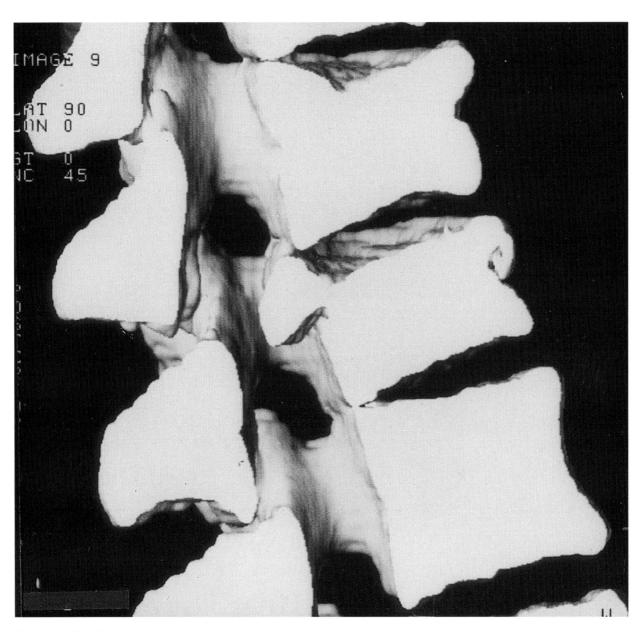

Figure 5.27 Three-dimensional CT of osteoporotic vertebral crush fractures (lateral view). Courtesy of Siemens AG, Erlangen, Germany

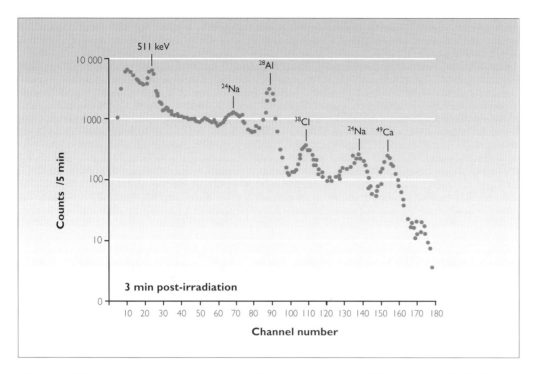

Figure 5.28 γ-Ray spectrum accumulated from a patient over 20 min starting 2–3 min after neutron activation. The peak from ^{49}Ca is clearly seen as well as those of other induced radionuclides. From reference 176, with permission

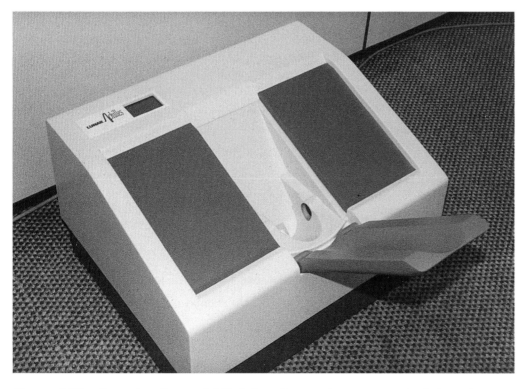

Figure 5.29 Apparatus (Lunar Achilles) for ultrasound measurement of the calcaneum. Courtesy of Lunar, Madison, WI

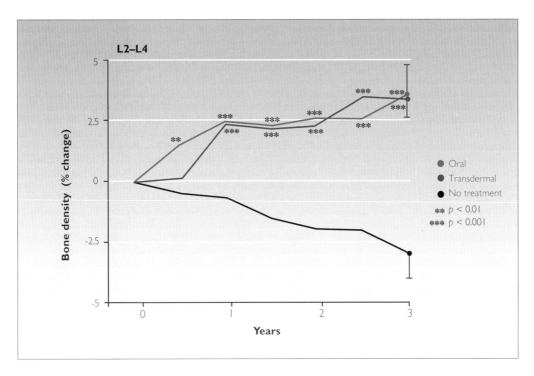

Figure 6.1 Changes in spine (L2–L4) bone density with oral and transdermal estrogen therapy compared with no estrogen treatment From reference 198, with permission

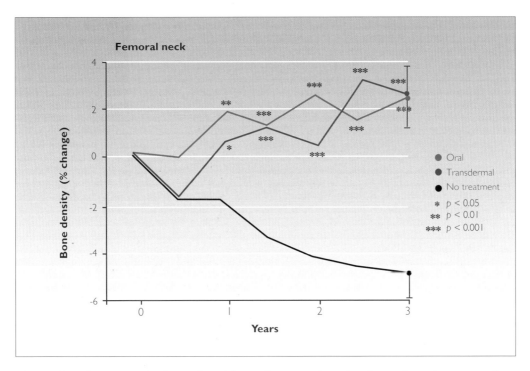

Figure 6.2 Changes in the femoral neck bone density with oral and transdermal estrogen therapy compared with no estrogen treatment From reference 198, with permission

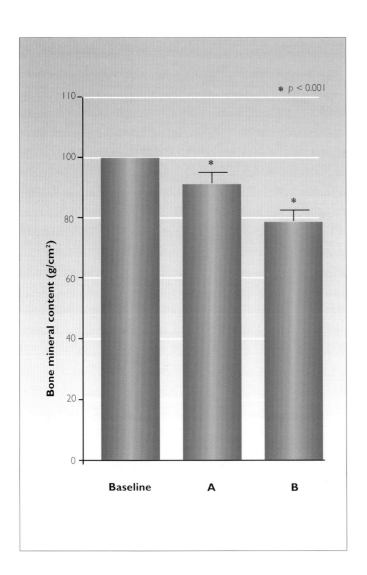

Figure 6.3 Prolonged effect of HRT following withdrawal of treatment. Bone density, as measured by SPA in the distal radius, is expressed as the initial percentage value (± SEM) in 242 healthy postmenopausal women at baseline and after 12 years. Group A (*n* = 68) received HRT for a mean of 5.4 years followed by a period off treatment; group B (*n* = 177) received no treatment for 12 years. *$p < 0.001$. From reference 200, with permission

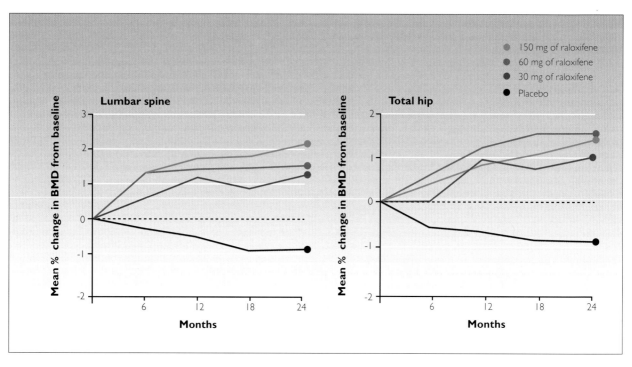

Figure 6.4 Bone mineral density (BMD) of the lumbar spine and total hip increased significantly ($p < 0.001$) with all dosage levels of raloxifene. From reference 205, with permission

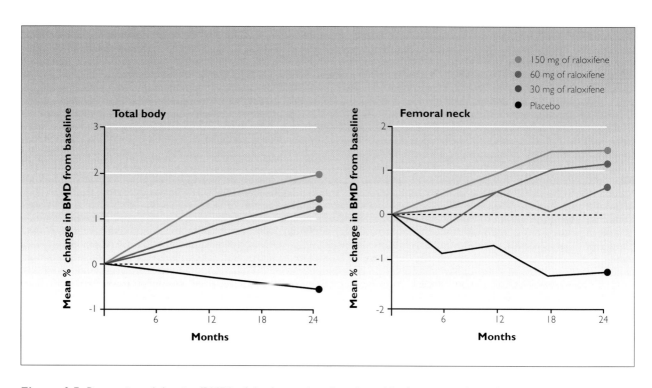

Figure 6.5 Bone mineral density (BMD) of the femoral neck and total body increased significantly ($p < 0.001$) with all dosage levels of raloxifene. From reference 205, with permission

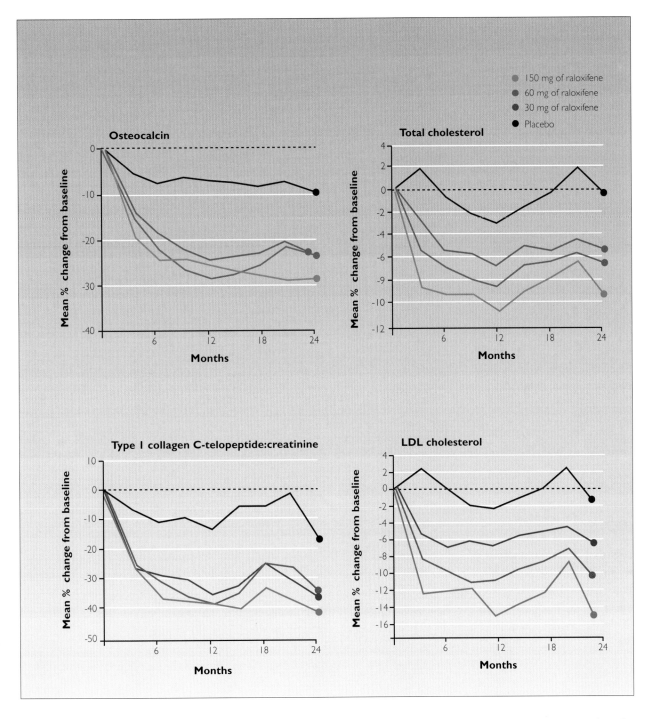

Figure 6.6 Markers of bone turnover were significantly decreased by all dosage levels of raloxifene compared to the placebo group as were total and LDL cholesterol. From reference 205, with permission

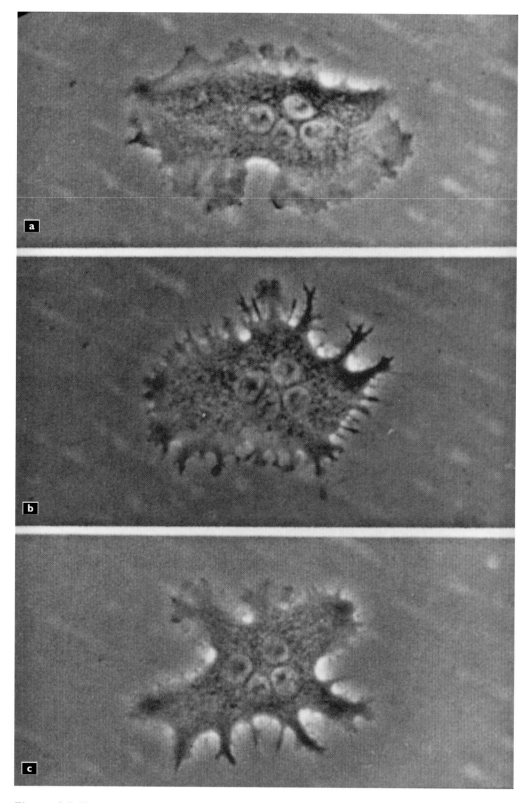

Figure 6.7 Time-lapse sequence of SEMs shows the response of an isolated osteoclast to calcitonin at time 0 (A), 10 min (B) and 120 min (C). From Stevenson JC, ed. *New Techniques in Metabolic Bone Disease*. London: Wright, 1990:63–81, with permission

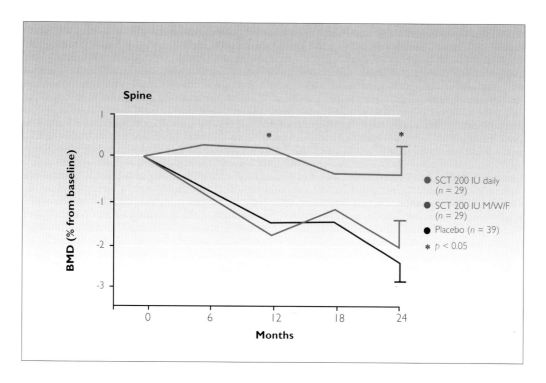

Figure 6.8 Percentage changes in spine bone mineral density (BMD) with salmon calcitonin (SCT) 200 IU daily compared with 200 IU three times a week and placebo over 2 years. From reference 217, with permission

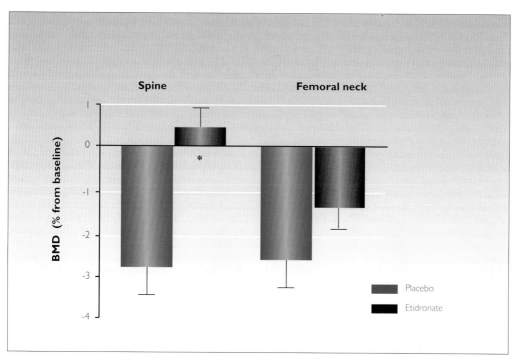

Figure 6.9 Mean percentage changes (± SEMs) in spine and femoral neck bone mineral density (BMD) from baseline in patients receiving etidronate compared with placebo for 12 months. The difference between the groups was statistically significant (*$p < 0.05$). From reference 221, with permission

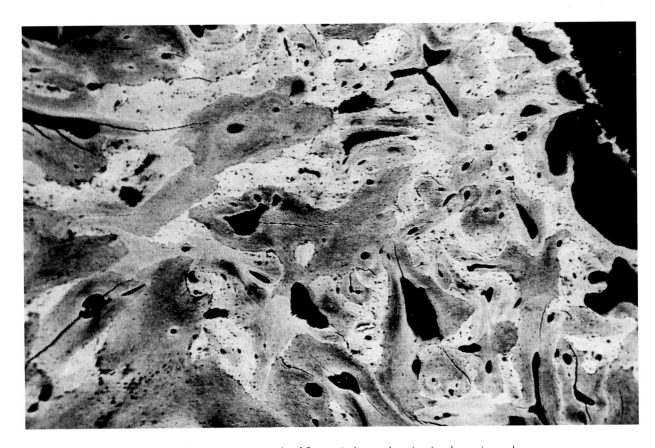

Figure 6.10 Back-scattered electron micrograph of fluorotic bone showing its dense irregular pattern. Courtesy of Professor Alan Boyde

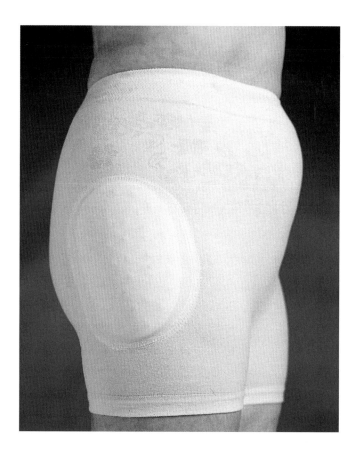

Figure 6.11 Hip protectors with rigid inserts have proved useful in preventing hip fracture in at-risk subjects. Courtesy of Robinson Healthcare, Chesterfield, UK

Index